Praise for *The Other Side of Bipolar*

"This book will give hope to those that feel hopeless and shine a light into the dark of how being different is difficult and made wrong. Hope does exist."

—GARY DOUGLAS
Author of *The Place*

"Lauren Polly leverages her triumphs, trials and life experience to show the reader how to create life on their own terms. A truly inspiring story with a revolutionary outlook on mental illness."

—JIM BRITT AND JIM LUTES
Creators of *The Change* Book Series

"It's not often that a book filled with such helpful tools and guidance reads like page-turning poetic fiction. If you have ever felt lost, *The Other Side of Bipolar* is truly in a 'must read' genre of its own."

—DR. DAIN HEER
Author of *Being You, Changing the World*

"Lauren Polly's book is a great contribution to what our world truly could be, if people know what gift they truly are and start enjoying their difference. Lauren Polly is gracefully shedding light on mental illness and what could be created beyond it. She uses her personal experience and shows the reader a different possibility."

—SUSANNA MITTERMAIER
Clinical Psychologist, Author and
Founder of Pragmatic Psychology

"Being diagnosed with a mental disorder can be devastating and crush a person's sense of self-worth. Lauren's raw and vulnerable tale of her own journey through the tortured world of mental illness inspires the reader to consider the possibility that what we've been labeling as disabilities may in fact be brilliant capacities unacknowledged. Lauren's triumph over her diagnosis challenges the current medical paradigm and is truly an invitation to a different reality with mental illness."

—ADRIANA POPESCU
Ph.D. Licensed Clinical Psychologist

"The kind of book you read in one sitting because the words are so compelling and the heroine someone you simply must see find her way." —BLOSSOM BENEDICT, International Speaker

"*The Other Side of Bipolar* sits apart from other autobiographical surveys of psychological struggles, offering readers the rare opportunity to explore and utilize many of the gifts formerly identified as disabilities. Any who have faced such a diagnosis will find this an inspiring, engrossing saga which offers hope, revelation, and much food for thought as it follows a journey that takes the identification of 'bipolar' and turns it upside down."

Anyone who wants a clear roadmap to a better approach will find *The Other Side of Bipolar* an engrossing, essential portrait of one woman who learned about mental health empowerment and how to reclaim hope. What can be expected from life after this process? There's no better indicator of all the possibilities than *The Other Side of Bipolar.*"

—DIANE DONAVON
Senior Reviewer, Midwest Book review

The Other Side of Bipolar

THE
OTHER SIDE
—— *of* ——
BIPOLAR

**Revealing Your Strengths to
Move Beyond the Diagnosis**

Lauren Polly

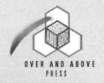

OVER AND ABOVE
PRESS

Published by Over And Above Press
Over and Above Creative Group
Los Angeles, CA
overandabovecreative.com

Editor: Lois Rose and Rick Benzel
Cover and Book Design: Susan Shankin & Associates
Cover and Author Photographer: Evelina Pentcheva

First edition
Library of Congress Control Number: 2016903587
ISBN: 978-0-9971077-0-8
Printed at Bang Printing in the United States of America
10 9 8 7 6 5 4 3 2 1
Distributed by SCB Distributors

Publisher's Cataloging-In-Publication Data
(Prepared by The Donohue Group, Inc.)
Names: Polly, Lauren.

Title: The other side of bipolar : revealing your strengths to move beyond the diagnosis / Lauren Polly.

Description: First edition. | Los Angeles, CA : Over And Above Press, [2016]
Identifiers: LCCN 2016903587 | ISBN 978-0-99710770-8 |
ISBN 978-0-99710771-5 (ebook)

Subjects: LCSH: Polly, Lauren. | Manic-depressive persons--Psychology. | Manic-depressive illness--Popular works. | Manic-depressive illness--Alternative treatment.

Classification: LCC RC516 .P65 2016 (print) | LCC RC516 (ebook) | DDC 616.895--dc23

Dedicated to those who know more is possible than what they have been told they can have and be.

Contents

Expressions of Gratitude   *xv*

INTRODUCTION   XVII

You're Not Alone   *xix*

PART 1: REVEALING CRAZY   1

1. LIFE GETS TOO LOUD   3

Am I Crazy?   *3*

Cabaret   *4*

Sideways but Straight   *5*

The Party   *6*

The Snake   *8*

Memory   *11*

My Award-Winning Performance   *12*

My Safe Haven   *14*

2. WHO CAN HELP ME NOW?   17

   Whispers in the Wind   *17*

   Kneeling to God   *18*

   The Bible Comes Alive   *20*

   The Chosen One   *21*

   Doesn't God Hear Me?   *23*

3. DARKNESS CREEPS IN   25

   The Thunderstorm   *25*

   Fight Dark with Dark   *27*

   Friend or Foe?   *28*

   The Smoky Quartz   *30*

   I'm Not Alone Anymore   *32*

   Savannah   *34*

   Dancing with Knives   *35*

4. THE DIAGNOSIS   39

   The Final Straw   *39*

   I Want Out   *40*

   Farewell Letter   *40*

   Discovery   *41*

   The Turning Point   *45*

   The "Oh" Moment   *49*

   Floating   *55*

   Drive to the Mental Hospital   *57*

5. BEING COMMITTED: TO BIPOLAR   59

   Reattachment of My Umbilical Cord   *59*

   A Night at the Movies   *60*

Learning My New Role   62

It's Not Safe to Share   66

6. COCKTAIL PARTY   69

My Body Is Angry   69

My Body: A Prison   72

My Body: A Pressure Cooker   74

My Body: A Pincushion   76

Losing What I Love the Most   76

My Body: Of Interest   77

The Crash   79

7. MY TURN TO CHOOSE   81

This Isn't Right   81

Dr. B's Recommendation   83

The Specialist   84

I Get to Choose   86

PART 2: REVEALING BRILLIANCE   89

8. SEARCHING FOR MY PLACE   91

The Yo-Yo Semester   91

Failed Launch   96

Flying to Fantasy Land   99

Holistic Psychiatry   102

The Shrink Who Changed Everything   104

9. I DON'T BELONG HERE   107

Dream Home   107

Reality Bites   109

My Break for Freedom 113

Scrapbooking Myself Together 116

10. LIVING FROM THE NECK UP 121

Brains Over Body 121

I Knew You Could Do This! 123

Time to Grow Up 125

My Mind vs. the Yoga Instructor 128

My Body: A Pressure Cooker Again 129

I Can Do This! 131

Paving the Way for Kids (Before I Have a Husband) 133

11. COMING HOME TO MY BODY 137

The Mind Has a Heart 137

Naked Yoga 140

Silence Inside and Out 143

A Name for the Dark Energies 145

The Snake Reappears 146

12. ME? POWERFUL? 149

Peru 149

The Whispers Return 150

It's Just Me Again 155

The Healer Speaks 156

Moon Light Ritual Bath 160

13. YOU MEAN I'M NOT CRAZY? 163

Is it Time? 163

The Payoff 165

I Don't Belong in a Box 168

You Are a Very Powerful Woman   169
You're Not Crazy—You're Remembering   171

14. RECLAIMING ALL OF ME   175
    Exploration   175
    The Book Comes Alive Again   180
    Ghosts   183
    The (Past-Life) Walk   186
    Is It Mine? Or Someone Else's?   189
    It's Not Mine!   193

15. NEW POSSIBILITIES   195
    Coming Home   195
    Bubbles of Pleasure   197
    Life Is Different Now   200
    Caged Animal   203
    Breaking Free   205
    Rose Garden   209
    I've Come a Long Way   210
    A Final Note to You, Dear Reader...   213
    Resources   215

ABOUT THE AUTHOR   217

WORKSHOPS   218
    Access Bars®   218
    Access Foundation®   218
    Talk to the Entities®   219
    Being Social   219
    Happy Body Happy You   220
    Mental Health Empowerment   220

Expressions of Gratitude

MY FAMILY
*For giving me roots while always encouraging me
to spread my wings and fly*

DR. JOHN TATUM
*For planting the seeds of success and
lighting a new path for me*

DR. ADRIANA POPESCU
*For being the first to acknowledge that I was never crazy.
I was remembering. And there is a difference.*

GARY DOUGLAS
*For pioneering a set of tools that allowed me
to create the life I always knew was possible*

DR. DAIN HEER
*For showing me how to change the cacophony
of the world into a symphony of possibilities*

SHANNON O'HARA
For emboldening me to be present with what I know

MEGAN WALROD
For being my book angel

Introduction

I WAS DIAGNOSED WITH BIPOLAR when I was fourteen, after a suicide attempt. What followed was sixteen years of being drugged, disempowered, and made wrong by others and myself. I was in constant fear that I would be put away in a mental institution. I exhausted myself trying to be normal so I could fit in with a world that told me I was crazy. I watched my family struggle to find ways to help me.

I was on multiple medications for six years before a doctor even mentioned the roles that stress management, diet, exercise and self-awareness could play in my recovery. I weaned myself off fourteen pills a day (my all-time high: no pun intended) down to nothing with the support of some very forward-thinking doctors and self-help techniques.

It was another three years after getting off all the meds before I gained a radical and unique perspective on my diagnosis: rather than judging myself as wrong I began to see my 'disabilities' as gifts and capacities that had been misunderstood. Discovering this new perspective changed my life. I stopped making myself wrong, constantly editing myself, and trying to be 'normal' so I could fit in. I started exploring and accessing more of my innate gifts that allow me to be more fully who I am while contributing to the world in joyful and satisfying ways.

If you have been recently diagnosed, or have lived with a diagnosis for most of your life, I wrote this book for you. If you're anything like I was, you have judged yourself, made yourself wrong, and struggled to make sense of what it means to be "bipolar" or to have "PTSD" or "name that diagnosis." Also like me, you've sensed another perspective beyond what the medical system knows. You just haven't found it, yet.

Even if you've never had a diagnosis but have always felt different, as though you don't fit in anywhere—I wrote this book for you, too. Chances are, also like me, you have judged yourself for your difference and judged others for not "getting" you. You have hid your uniqueness by conforming to those around you. Or you have rebelled against others to prove you're not like them. Either way, you feel isolated and alone, your difference its own kind of disability. Just as I did, you have withdrawn from the world, seeking refuge in living a small existence. But you desire more. You sense another possibility beyond the struggle. You just haven't found it yet, either.

This book tells my story of discovering the other side of bipolar and moving beyond a diagnosis. I share my journey with you to show you another possibility beyond the wrongness of your diagnosis and your difference. So that you, too, can explore your 'disability' as a gift, and discover the magic and beauty of who you truly are.

Will you join me on the journey?

You're Not Alone

I FELT CRAZY and alone during the years I lived with a diagnosis of bipolar. I wished someone had wrapped their arms around me and said to me the words I now share with you . . .

You're not alone.

I know it seems like the end; like it isn't worth it to keep going. As if there is nothing on the other side of this pain, embarrassment, shame, anger and confusion you feel. That you can't possibly survive it. The sadness is suffocating. The confusion can spin your head. You may feel like you are losing grip on reality. That you are going crazy. That there is something really wrong with you.

Try as you may, you cannot shut out the pain. It is hard to see past it. It seems that it will never get better—that there is no hope.

You may think the world will be better off without you. You may think that you are so insignificant that your absence will not be missed, that life will go on and no one will even remember you.

But what if you are important beyond measure?

What if your absence will rob the world of what only you can offer it?

What if the bullies, the judgmental people, the hate and sadness in this world aren't more real or true than your kindness, gentleness and hope?

I am here to let you know there is a possibility for your life far beyond what you can see right now. There is freedom from this pain.

— PART 1 —
Revealing Crazy

1

Life Gets too Loud

AM I CRAZY?

BUBBLY JOY GROWS FROM INSIDE. It doesn't seem to fit in my body. The expansion is too much, too powerful and too unfamiliar. It's going to explode.

I have to get outside. NOW. I need to run it off. The house isn't big enough to contain me. I'm suffocating and at any moment the vibration from my body will move to the house and down it will come.

I get outside, into the open. I run and the energy that felt so suffocating inside now takes flight. I expand more, getting bigger and bigger. I feel my ribcage bursting—or is that my heart?

In one breath the earth enters me from my feet and ripples through my body. I've got goose bumps on my arms and my hair is standing on end. The sky touches my head and invades my brain. The trees and plants draw closer to me.

I can't find my body anymore. I CAN'T FIND MY BODY ANYMORE! I am larger than the earth; the earth is inside of me, our hearts beating as one. I am no longer running but skipping. My arms and hair are flying; my feet barely touching the grass.

And then, like a deer suddenly aware of the hunter's intense gaze, I stop in my tracks. I look to the left and meet the shocked gaze of two classmates playing soccer nearby. My mind is flooded with noise I hear the words, "Crazy," "Strange," and "Wrong," as though they're screaming them at me, but their mouths are closed.

That's not true, is it? But it's in my head and sounds like my voice. Am I crazy?

CABARET

I TAKE MY PLACE on stage, the sequins my mom sewed onto my skirt for my 8th grade dance recital flashing in the light, my lavender leotard soft against my skin.

I hold still, listening to *"Cabaret."* The music pulses through me and moves me around the stage.

I imagine all the Broadway dancers who ever danced to this song moving with me across the floor. The stage lights blind me and block out the sight of all the people watching me, but I can feel their gaze like gentle caresses on my skin. I feel them joining me in the churning waves of the dance.

The music continues to build and swell. A giggle wiggles up from my belly. The waves of music stir up the familiar bubbles of energy. I let the bubbles lead the way, guiding me from one move to the next.

The last chord of the music hits and I strike my final pose. I pause, feeling the beat of the music still coursing through my body. I bow and hear the thundering applause.

The applause fades away and I look up and see the familiar walls of the basement, with the foosball tables and couches pushed to the side. The flash of the sequins in the mirror catches my eye. I turn and gaze at my image, tracing my hands along the curves where my costume folds around me. Where do I end and where does the costume begin?

I giggle. I turn and look around the basement again. This is my stage. My sanctuary.

SIDEWAYS BUT STRAIGHT

ALTHOUGH THE HEAT OF the day has gone, the air is still warm on my bare skin. It is so thick it sticks and presses to me like a full body embrace. The wind picks up and brushes against my body with soft gentle strokes. I sigh and smile. I notice the tickling sensation of bubbles in my belly.

The stars above twinkle and I watch them dancing. I giggle as I feel the same dancing energy inside. The bubbles expand.

I look around at my companions: my brother, Drew, is here, along with other teenagers from a visiting youth group. Today is the first time I've met them. I look back behind our group and see my parents strolling hand in hand. They brought us all here to Washington D.C. for a day of sightseeing.

Being surrounded by the people who know me the most and those who do not know me at all is oddly comforting and freeing at the same time. I wonder to myself . . . Who would I like to be now?

I become bigger somehow. The space around me opens up. The more it opens up the bigger I get. The bubbles intensify and build as well. They spread up and out my arms and legs. Now I can see the entire city: streets empty of cars, massive monuments lit up, other tourists taking in the sights.

The night feels important and grand. I stretch my arms overhead taking up even more space. The bubbles keep growing and the space around me keeps expanding.

We're all laughing and joking. I'm being a "dumb blond," as I've discovered people really seem to like when I act ditzy. So I sing out loud, *"I am e-f-f-e-r-v-e-s-c-e-n-t! That's the only way I know how to spell it!"* and everyone laughs.

As we laugh, walk and play, the bubbles keep building. The energy of everyone's laughter lifts me up. The bubbles take over. I explode.

I twist my body suddenly to face sideways but I keep walking in a straight line. *"Ha! I'm going sideways but straight!"* I sing out really loud. It seems very obvious and dumb but funny at the same time. Everyone laughs and copies me. The entire group begins walking sideways but straight and singing, *"Sideways but straight!"* We walk up the Lincoln Memorial steps *sideways but straight* so amused by our cleverness.

My new friends laugh harder and harder. It's fun at first. But then the laughter gets too loud and presses in on my ears, my body. The bubbles burst and fade. I look around: everyone is still laughing and looking to me. I don't want to disappoint them so I put on a smile and keep doing it, forcing the motions that were only a moment ago so fun and easy.

THE PARTY

IT'S NEW YEAR'S EVE. There's music playing in the background as my parents, Drew and I get the house ready for our neighbors' arrival. We've had a party every New Year's Eve for as long as I can remember. I love getting dressed up, decorating the house and playing hostess with my parents.

Our neighbors begin arriving in small groups of two or more, each carrying a dish to share. It's my job to take their gift of food and place it on the long dining room table. I enjoy seeing all the colors and textures of the different food. I sneak a small taste of each before heading out to the entryway again to greet the next round of people.

I skip around and greet everyone with a wide smile. The ticklish feeling of the soda pop bubbles fills my belly just like they did that day in D.C.

The house fills with a buzz as more neighbors arrive. It's like one by one another instrument gets added to the orchestra. But this orchestra is out of tune with instruments that don't complement each other. The bubbles that had been happily floating around begin to churn.

All of a sudden the buzz grows so loud my bubbles burst and fizzle. My ears hurt and everything gets blurry. The voices around me collide with one another and cut like glass on my skin. The bouts of laughter are especially sharp.

While moments ago I had welcomed the attention from neighbors I greeted, now their questions and holiday cheer feel like a pillow being pushed against my face. I gasp for air. What's happening?

I start looking for quiet and empty space but it is difficult to find in this swirling crowd of people. Everyone I pass smiles and tries to talk to me but my voice goes away and I find it hard to respond to their questions.

What's wrong with me? Everyone else is having fun. Nobody else seems bothered by this out-of-tune orchestra.

I twist and turn as I make my way through the crowd, trying to keep space between each lump of people and myself. As I pass each group I'm caught up in different currents. I'm not sure how to navigate them.

Everyone appears jovial and in the "holiday spirit", but as I slide along the wall to pass by a group of three women chattering, I feel my belly and jaw clenching. I'm hit with a rush of anger. Yet all I see are smiles on their faces. What I see is not what I feel. Is what I'm feeling wrong? What's going on here?

I duck my head down and slip quietly behind the older woman who lost her husband this year. A wave of sadness drenches me and I wonder if it will take me down. Somehow I keep moving forward.

I gasp for breath. I become more and more confused as each person tries to engage with me. Do I respond to their words or the wave of emotion flowing through them and into me? Nobody else seems to be aware of these undercurrents.

Is it real or am I crazy?

THE SNAKE

EVERYONE IS TALKING ABOUT ME. Their voices whisper and whirl just out of earshot like the hum of a washing machine. My skin is on fire from their stares.

I walk through the hallways with my head down, heading for the cafeteria. I feel them watching me the same way animals stalk their prey: bonding together to take down a weaker species with the strength of the group. That's what I feel like—a different species.

I used to get along so well my classmates. I used to be happy. I used to laugh and have friends. What happened this year? When did I become the target?

I hide as much as I can. I hear people talking about how pretty I am. I attract attention even though I'm trying to avoid it. Somehow I laugh too loud. I smile too big. I'm too animated. I walk differently.

The attention I used to enjoy now feels dangerous. I can sense people picking me apart and now I do the same. "Be smaller," I tell myself. "Don't smile as much." "Don't laugh that loud."

My stomach tightens as I near the big wooden doors of the cafeteria. I hate this place. The noise of everyone reverberates off the walls and shakes my brain. I've taken to eating lunch in a teacher's classroom.

But there is no avoiding this place today. We are gathering for our 8th grade exams. The cafeteria has been re-organized to fit the entire class of 200 people.

As I pull open the door I see they've set up assigned seating. Thank God, at least I don't have to try to find someone to sit with. I head over to the other kids whose last names start with "P." My shoulders slump more as I see my tablemates. Popular kids. Mean kids. The whisperers.

I slide into my seat without even pulling out the chair. I don't want the scraping of the chair on the floor to alert them to my arrival. But I feel their eyes on me anyway. I keep my head down and hold my breath, worried that my fast breathing will attract more attention.

I turn my sharpened #2 pencil over and over in my hands, pretending to check the sharpness. Pretending to be deeply involved in something. Pretending to not notice them looking at me and then back and forth at each other.

The teacher comes to the table and holds out the test packet for me. I lean over to take it and as I do my hand curls up awkwardly in a claw-like shape facing the ceiling. I hear a giggle and look to my left. I see a girl at the next table with her hand in the same position as mine was. Is she mimicking me? I quickly lean back in my chair and bring both hands down under the table on my lap.

I glance to my right and see two other girls smiling widely at each other. Are they smiling about me? Are they copying my grin like they've done before? How can I sit so that everyone leaves me alone?

If I were a magician I would make myself disappear.

That's when I see something out of the corner of my eye. A stream of smoke curling and slithering its way around and over the tables. A smoky snake. I sit spellbound. Frozen in fear. I know it's here for me. It's coming to get me just like all the other kids.

I hear its "sssss" in my ears and I recognize this hatred: it's the pinpricks that make my skin crawl as I walk through the hallways. It's the fire starter that makes me blush red constantly whenever a small bit of attention is directed my way. It's the disapproving voice that makes me lower my eyes to the floor. It's what wants me to disappear. It only lasts a second and is gone.

I shake my head quickly and focus on the test. My grades have slipped a lot this year since I've been so busy trying to hide. I can't risk getting a low score on this test. I spend all my energy blocking out the other kids—it's easier now that their attention is wrapped up in the test also.

The test is long and hard. We all breathe a sigh of relief as we turn in our papers. I catch one of my tablemate's eyes briefly as I hand her my paper. She smiles kindly at me. I almost cry and release a big wave of breath. It's been so long since I've sensed kindness here. But just like the smoky slithering snake, it evaporates in an instant. Was it ever there in the first place?

Mr. D. waddles up to a microphone that's been placed in the front of the room. He's a large man and the students giggle at him as he moves heavily across the floor. My heart thuds in my chest and I look down feeling sorry for him. I know what it's like to receive unwanted attention.

"We have the results of the elections for the student counselors. We had asked you all to write the name of classmates who you felt would be good leaders and would be able to be trained as peer counselors for you. Here are the 5 you all picked."

His voice is hard to listen to as it bounces back and forth between the walls of the cafeteria. Even the linoleum floor seems to be reverberating with it. My hands instinctively cover my ears and I close my eyes, tired of trying to focus over the stares and whispers of my classmates.

I can feel hundreds of pinpricks on my skin. My body flushes red and starts to shake under the force of it. I open my eyes and stop breathing: everyone is staring at me. There is applause, which just adds to the noise in my head. I fight the urge to run out of the room.

"Stand up, Lauren. You were elected," says the girl sitting next to me. The one who had smiled so kindly at me.

I rise slowly to my feet but I can't feel the floor. My long, strong dancer legs tremble and shake as my breath comes in short spurts. I've performed in front of crowds since I was 3. What is going on with me?

I see the smoke snake curling off to my left. A quiet hiss is added to the thunder-like sound of the applause. I sit down quickly. I was elected. I didn't volunteer myself. It was an open ballot.

I look around suspiciously at my classmates who I know hate me. What's the joke they are all in on now? It's bigger than I thought. Everyone in here is in on it. I wonder if the teachers are too. The hissing becomes louder.

What is real and what isn't?

MEMORY

I MOVE SLOWLY DOWN the stairs, my ballet shoes in hand. It's about 4:30. School is over, homework is done, and it's time to dance. The basement is dark, dank and damp, like a dungeon.

I plop onto the beanbag by the stereo and drop my shoes. I feel so heavy it's hard to breathe.

I fumble through the records, looking for one that matches my mood. *"Memory"* from Cats jumps out to me. I love this song: its melody filled with regret and longing is just what I need. I put the record on and hit play. I close my eyes as the music fills me up. There are not waves strong enough to move my body tonight.

The murky dimness of the basement fills my mind. I feel like I'm sinking in water. I let the heaviest parts of my body fall off so I can rise up and breathe again. I sigh. The music moves through me.

I return to the heaviness of my body. I'm still sitting in the same position: cross-legged on the beanbag. I look at the clock. It's 7:30. The basement is quiet, *"Memory"* having long stopped playing. Where did I go? I look around the basement: it doesn't look like a dungeon or a stage.

A part of me wants to know where I went, but it can't fight this dullness all around me. I shrug my shoulders. It doesn't really matter. I gather up my body, as though I'm carrying a bag of bricks that gets heavier and heavier as I walk up the stairs.

I pause at the top of the steps and take a deep breath. I plaster a smile on my face: it's time to return to the real world. I whisper to myself, "I'm not crazy. I didn't do anything weird. I'm okay," and open the door.

MY AWARD-WINNING PERFORMANCE

IT'S ALMOST THE END of the day. I'm almost free. I keep crossing and uncrossing my legs, shifting in my seat from side to side. My eyes watch the clock. Tick tick tick closer to 3 p.m. when I can leave this hell they call a school.

The whooshing of the whispers is so loud now that white noise is constantly present. My head hurts. My eyes stay on the clock unable to tolerate even one more stare. One more whisper would be too much. I think if I can just hold out until 3 p.m. then I could find a quiet place to cry. Maybe if I keep focused on the clock then I can keep myself from breaking down in front of people.

The snake circles. The pinpricks of eyes poke at me, burning my skin and making it flush. But I don't look at anyone. I just watch the clock.

Finally the bell rings. I stand up quickly to sprint from the room, but my teacher calls me over to her desk. She's a favorite of mine. Easy to talk to and kind, but I'm in no mood to chat today. Her eyes are concerned.

"Lauren, I'm here if you ever need to talk about anything. Anything at all." I can't even speak. Her worry makes me worry. Is it so bad that she notices the whispers also? Have I become that big of a target?

I nod my head slowly. "Ok" squeaks out, barely audible over the whooshing in my mind. I turn and leave quickly. Her concern makes the tears harder to hold in. Luckily the bathroom is close by. I lock myself inside the yellow stall just as tears break free and fall.

I don't stay long. I can't afford to. The bus will leave soon and I don't want anyone to know I'm upset, that they have had an effect on me. I splash water on my face, take a deep breath and make myself as numb as possible. The bus is loud as always. The trees are calming and help me tune it out as we drive past them.

Mom's waiting for me when I get home. Today I have an early dance class and she's there to take me. I breathe deeply as I near the garage door leading into the house. I can't let her know.

It's too embarrassing. I hate myself for being unpopular, I hate myself for having other people hate me, I hate myself for being what I am: an easy target.

"Hi Tuey," she calls out from the kitchen using my childhood nickname. I smile as I see her warm hazel eyes. I wish others could see me the way she does. It feels so good to have someone light up at the sight of me. My heart swells up and my eyes water.

No. No tears. I won't let her see. I won't let any of that crap come into my home. I won't be unsafe and sad here too. I shove the tears down and force a smile. All the roles I've played in theater performances are paying off. Playing the role of Lauren—an encore of the happy days—is something I am quite good at.

No. No one here needs to know.

MY SAFE HAVEN

I DON'T WANT TO be around people. They are too loud. I drag myself up the stairs to my room. My bones must be made of lead, my muscles of sand bags. When did I get so tired? When did I get so heavy?

I step into my room and close the door quietly behind me. There is no washing machine whoosh of whispers here. No hissing of the smoky snake stalking me. No sharp noises to jostle my brain and hurt my head.

I sigh. I'm safe. For now.

Soft golden light dances through the peach curtains. It warms me and comforts my eyes after the stares and fluorescent lights at school. Even though it's not nighttime and I'll need to get my dance clothes on in an hour to head to class, I put on my silk nightie. The material is soft and soothing.

I pull back the comforter and slide onto the sheets. I arrange two pillows to press into my back and curl around two pillows in front of me. I feel cradled and held. I melt into the pillows, exhausted from the effort of protecting myself from the stares and whispers at school.

Everything used to be so vivid and alive to me, but now it's all gray. I close my eyes and welcome the darkness.

---- 2 ----

Who Can Help Me Now?

WHISPERS IN THE WIND

DANCE CLASS IS OVER. I leave the chatter of the studio to wait out front for my mom. As I step outside into the early fall sunshine I smile at the red, orange and yellow leaves painting the trees lining the street. I wander down the sidewalk in front of the other stores, relaxing into an easy sway of walking. There are no fixed movements out here like there are in the studio.

The wind picks up and I pause and turn to it. The sun warms my face and the wind strokes my arms. As I breathe in I feel the wind: it moves beneath my skin and swirls through my body. It's not like those whispers at school, and I like it.

I feel a gentle tug. Something is pulling me forward. Whispery soft sounds breathe into my ears. The hairs on my arms rise up. Who is talking to me? What do they want me to see?

I feel the anticipated arrival of my mom. *"I should turn back,"* shoots through my mind. However, I continue down the sidewalk with the wind. I reach the end of the strip mall and see the railroad tracks that lie beyond it. I see several big blue dumpsters at the backs of the stores. Nobody is around. Again I feel the tug of Mom's imminent arrival, but I keep moving forward.

The whispers seem to be calling me towards the tracks themselves. Flashes of being hit by an oncoming train flicker so fast through me that I almost don't catch them. My heart starts to pound. I shake my head and stop abruptly.

What am I doing? I cover my heart with my hands. I pause and listen intently. The whispers are gone now. I can only feel a slight stirring in my belly. I turn around. The wind at my back now pushes me towards Mom.

I return along the sidewalk quickly and spot her waiting in the car. As we drive away I look back at the railroad tracks. As the metal of the tracks shines in the sunlight I feel the faintest hint of a stir within me. I shake my head again to clear out any of those whispers and make sure they don't travel home with me. They are not allowed there.

KNEELING TO GOD

I SINK INTO MY favorite chair in the corner of my room, resting into the curves of its sage-green-and-peach-covered arms. The house is quiet. It's past my bedtime, but I can't sleep. The brass lamp beside me casts a soft glow of light, pooling on the heavy book in my lap as if spotlighting this moment . . . the first time I am opening my own Bible.

I rest my hands on the soft, brown leather and close my eyes. I see an image of my family sitting together on the red-covered cushions that line the pews in the new church we've been going to for the past month. It was Mom who led the way for us to return to church. Now, though we don't talk about God at home very much and don't read from the Bible together, there's a sense that we're all being looked after.

The heavy Bible sitting on my lap was a gift from my parents. I had asked for it after I noticed that everyone at church had one. I can hear the pastor's words ring in my ear as he talked about the power of the book and its connection to God, "He is always with you. He is always watching you. You can look to His Book for answers and guidance."

Suddenly I'm back at school: the stares, the hissing snake, the whispers. I shake my head quickly. The pictures fade but they leave behind a heavy mixed up feeling inside. It's hard to breathe. I still hear the faintest hiss in the distance. I open my eyes and pick up the Bible, holding it between my hands. If anyone can help me it is God.

I open the Bible to the middle and land on a passage about salvation and asking for forgiveness. Is this a sign? Maybe I did something bad to deserve what's happening to me. I read the passage looking for a story of how I may be deserving of the ridicule, shame and embarrassment I am going through at school.

I don't find one immediately but am determined to keep looking. I want God to know I'm paying attention to His signs and messages. I wonder if I should start praying. A flash of Mom and Dad tucking me in and saying prayers with me when I was little runs through my mind. They were kneeling on the floor on either side of my bed. Maybe if I kneel too?

I stand up and lay the Bible on my chair. My bare knees sink into the carpet. I clasp my hands together and rest my elbows on the bed. I close my eyes and breathe deeply. "God, please. I'm sorry if I did something to upset you. Please make this stop. Please make people leave me alone. Please make the snake go away."

I open my eyes fast, expecting a flash of light or something spectacular. But I don't see anything. I crawl into bed with a sigh but also with a small glimmer of hope that something may change. I'll have to wait and see.

THE BIBLE COMES ALIVE

DAYS HAVE PASSED AND there's been no change. No improvement. No silence from the whispers. No peace from the smoky snake. It's past bedtime and I can't sleep, again. The Bible calls to me.

I sit in my favorite chair with my Bible. I flip it open, allowing God to take me where He wants me to go. This passage is dark. Murderous. Revenge-filled. What is He telling me with this one?

My stomach clenches and burns as I read. The passages are so real they pulsate on the page. The story of Cain and Abel wronging each other and the vengeance that God calls forth vibrates through me.

The story creeps into my fingers and up my arms. I begin to read out loud, taking on the voice of the wronged. The righteous anger moves in waves through my arms and fills my chest. I speak louder and louder as I continue on this harrowing journey with the characters. The anger spreads through my body and pools in my eyes. I see red.

The sound of my door bursting open and the whoosh of air from the hallway shock me out of the story and into my bedroom. The images of revenge are replaced with my brother standing in the doorway, the hallway light shining behind him.

"Are you okay?" he asks.

"I'm fine. Sorry I woke you up," I say in my normal pleasing voice.

He lingers for a second, looking at me with his gentle blue eyes. Then he closes the door softly. I close the Bible and put it down on the table by my chair. *"Please,"* I whisper, *"Please stay. Please stay in the Bible."*

I shake my arms, releasing the dark anger of the Bible brothers from my body. I crawl into bed without kneeling to pray. I put my hand on my stomach. I can still feel the story throbbing there. What just happened? A seed was planted in me. How do I get rid of it now?

THE CHOSEN ONE

THE SOUND FROM THE speakers fills the large room. It's soothing, very different from the voices in the cafeteria. Somehow I don't mind being in a room full of people at church.

I like the music. "Modern hymns" they are called; old lyrics with new beats and more instruments. It's jazzy and if you don't pay attention to the words you would never know you were singing to God. The lyrics are projected onto a large screen at the front of the church so we can sing along. The title flashes as the opening notes play. "Here I am Lord."

Yes, I think to myself, Lord here I am.

The first verse begins. My breath catches in my throat. The pulse jumps from the speakers into my body, pushing its way through like the Bible verses do. This pulse is different though—not dark and vengeful like the verses I've been reading. These verses are a call to action. A song about purpose. Will it show me my purpose?

My lips move to the words as I read them in time with the music. But my voice fades as I recognize that this song was written for me.

"I, the Lord of sea and sky
I have heard My people cry.
All who dwell in dark and sin,
My hand will save.

"I who made the stars of night,
I will make their darkness bright.
Who will bear My light to them?
Whom shall I send?

"Here I am Lord, Is it I Lord?
I have heard You calling in the night.
I will go Lord, if You lead me.
I will hold Your people in my heart."

The next verses flash on the screen. As I move my lips to
the words I almost cry. It describes exactly what I experience at
school. Relief and gratitude fill me as I melt into the music. The
waves come and I start to rock.

"I, the Lord of snow and rain,
I have born my people's pain.
I have wept for love of them, They turn away.
I will break their hearts of stone,
Give them hearts for love alone.
I will speak My word to them,
Whom shall I send?"

I find my voice for the second chorus. I sing out knowing I
can connect with God and maybe just maybe now He will listen
and respond.

"Here I am Lord, Is it I Lord?
I have heard You calling in the night.

I will go Lord, if You lead me.
I will hold Your people in my heart."

I get it now. I was sent here to show people the results of their mean actions. That is why I am getting picked on. I was sent here to break their hearts of stone like the song says. I am to be the sacrifice. I'm not crazy: I have been sent by God.

A wave of energy rises up through me as the last note of the song hangs in the air. I'm the Chosen One. God chose me.

How can I serve you Lord? Here I am . . .

DOESN'T GOD HEAR ME?

THE RELIEF OF KNOWING I'm not crazy, that I am the Chosen One, hasn't lasted long. People don't see me as a Chosen One. People are mean. I can't figure out how to break their hearts of stone. The world is dark. I feel even more isolated. The waves moving through me are so big now. I'm tired of the ups and downs.

Every night I read Bible passages and sing songs from church. But it is not enough. I start opening the window and speaking to the sky, sometimes even yelling to the heavens to make sure God hears me. But He doesn't respond. Can God not hear me? Or is He just choosing not to listen?

I climb out the window of my parent's bathroom onto the roof so I can be closer to Him. I pray and sing softly looking into the twinkling stars like I'm looking into the twinkle of His eye. But still no response.

Every passage read, every song sung, every word thrown into the night sky is a prayer to God, *"Please God. Please God. Save me."* I wake up every morning and listen closely for signs that God has fixed me. With all my praying and speaking to the sky I expect the noise in my head to go away, to be quiet. But it doesn't. Why isn't God helping me?

I keep reading the Bible at night and speaking to the sky. I go back and forth between the dark passages and more uplifting ones I learned in Youth Group. Back and forth, back and forth. Heavy and light. Ominous and filled with salvation.

Nothing changes. The seed in my belly throbs. The hissing snake curls closer to me every day. The whispers grow. The world pushes on me from all sides. I am squished and squashed, screaming silently.

I hate being a martyr, being the Chosen One. If this is my God-given purpose I want to give it back. It sucks. I can't take it anymore.

One Friday night I throw my Bible on the floor. This isn't working. God has abandoned me. I am not worthy of His rescue. The night sky is quiet. The house is quiet. There is nobody here to save me. God is not hearing my prayers, or worse, He doesn't care. I am worthless. I am completely on my own.

If God won't fix me or at least show me the purpose of what is going on with me, what's the point of sticking around? Why continue being in a world that is loud, uncaring and mean?

I want to curl up and go away. I don't want to be here anymore.

---------- 3 ----------

Darkness Creeps In

THE THUNDERSTORM

MORE WHISPERS. MORE LOOKS.

Scenes from the day at school flash through my mind as I wander from room to room in the house. Each scene is like a burst of fire, ready to burn me alive if I stand still for a moment. So I walk up and down the stairs, through each room, again and again. My skin itches. I run my fingernails down my milky white arms and watch red trails rise in their wake.

Suddenly there is a groan of thunder from the other side of the valley, almost like a battle cry. It's faint to my ears but I can feel the rumble deep in my belly. Ah, I smile. A storm is coming.

I move to the back screened-in porch. I step around the metal tables and chairs to stand right near the screen. This is one of my favorite spots: the screens provide protection from the elements and I can still have a full view of the storm rolling in over the forest.

The humidity is thick and calms me as it presses against me. I feel like someone is wrapping me in a giant bear hug. The wind picks up and swirls around me, caressing my skin and gently lifting my hair. I moan in pleasure and soften into the storm.

The wind slips inside of me and begins to stir up my thoughts. I'm startled. Usually when I'm this relaxed my head gets quiet. But now the struggles of the day swirl around my mind in a confusing flurry. The scenes are moving fast and make me dizzy. I shut my eyes and cover my ears with my hands but it is no use—they're inside of me.

I fight the urge to run away. No. No more running away. I take my hands off my ears and place them on my hips. I open my eyes wide and stare into the dense clouds overhead. I'm staring at God, meeting His cold gaze with steel.

Boiling hot rage rises up and out of me as the first of the heavy raindrops fall. The covered porch keeps the water from falling directly down on me but somehow that Son of a Bitch still gets me wet. The cold prickles hit me like He's spitting in my face, taunting me.

The rumble of the thunder He creates to stir and agitate is nothing compared to my own. Rolls of rage ripple through me, building up until my entire body is shaking. My storm is so big the porch and ground begin to shake too.

I have been praying for months for Him to fix this and no answer has come, no relief, no support. There has only been more intensity, more noise and more isolation. I'm *done*.

I grab a metal chair and sit facing the open woods. I keep staring at the sky, staring at God. God do your worst and your best. Send the lightning. Electricity bristles and zzzsssttt through my body. My chest explodes as I send out a red fireball of rage. He replies by lighting up the sky. I squint and shoot black bolts at Him. He cracks my ears with a loud *boom!*

This ends now.

I am invincible, equal to, and one with Him. We play off each other, grumble-flash, rumble-slash, building and colliding. Part of me is begging Him to take me out with a lightning bolt, but I know that He can't. Or won't.

Tears blur my vision. My rage storm dissolves as quickly as it came on. I am now weak, powerless and in need of Him. *Take me. Please take me.*

The door to the porch opens. "Lauren, what are you doing out here in the storm?" calls my mom.

The power that I was, taking on God, is gone. I'm just me again. I make my lips curl up in a smile and look up at my mom. No need to tell her anything. I get up from the chair and follow her into the house.

I pause at the doorway and take one final look at the sky. One last acknowledgment before I shut the door between us forever. Let's see how He likes being ignored.

FIGHT DARK WITH DARK

DARKNESS CREEPS INTO MY room as the sun sets. I reach up to turn on my reading lamp not taking my eyes off the page. As I turn on the light I notice my hips are stiff. I have been sitting here reading in the same spot since this morning. I stretch out my legs and then curl them back underneath me as I turn the page.

Just like the Bible brothers' story of revenge, this story pulsates through me. It creeps up my arms, into my chest and down into the dark seed in my belly. "Flowers in the Attic"—yes, precious flowers that have been locked away. Surviving against all odds. It's what I am too. I become the lead character and she becomes me.

Cathy Dollanganger is a dancer. I'm a dancer also. She is held captive by her mean stepmom and locked away in the attic. I'm locked in my own prison by my captors at school. She is denied food and wastes away. I am denied kindness and am wasting away. She is unsafe and never knows what will happen next. Neither do I. Her only solace is dancing. Mine too.

The angry seed planted by the story of the Bible brothers sparks and vibrates as I read. I press my hands to my stomach again just like I did the night I read the Bible. Just like I've been doing whenever I hear the whoosh of the whispers at school. Whenever I feel the pinpricks of eyes on me. Whenever I feel the terror of being hunted.

The snake's hiss of hatred softens in my ear and it backs off as I acknowledge the dark seed taking root. The message is clear: fight dark with dark. This book is right. So is the Bible. This is a cruel and unsafe world. My only hope is to find something to protect myself with.

FRIEND OR FOE?

MY HEAD SPINS WITH the white noise. I squirm in my skin and look around the classroom: everyone's eyes are down, pen to paper, focusing on their work. I can still hear whispers though. My belly clenches, in and out, in and out. The angry seed is irritated.

I claw my arm. My flesh rises in red gashes in protest. I hear a high-pitched squeak that grates every nerve, like nails on a chalkboard. The snake circles me, hissing loudly. *"Enough!"* I command it with my mind, not wanting to draw attention to me. I'm still studying the battlefield around me. I'm not ready to make my move just yet.

The smoky snake curls under my desk, listening, obeying, delighted that I am acknowledging it at last. Its role has begun changing along with my moods: from tormentor to friend; pest to pet; boss to servant; something to be feared, something to be loved.

Scenes of last period's theater class play in my mind: my loud laughter, the look of disgust a friend shot at me. Remembering her small eyes and grimace make the red marks on my arm pulse with heat. Her words, "You're annoying," sting in my chest.

Enemies surround me. Everywhere there is someone waiting to pounce on me. I've been quiet and good long enough. I'm done with being the victim. The dark seed hears this and thrusts cold hard steel up my spine in agreement. My breath sucks in as my spine straightens. I lift my chin up as waves of anger rip through me.

"Oh, they'll be sorry they messed with me."

"Yes, they'll be sorry they messed with us," agrees the snake.

The noise in my head gets louder. Thoughts get jagged and sharp. My head snaps sharply to the left at a whisper whoosh I hear from two girls giggling a few seats away. I feel my skin peeling back in protest, scalded by the heat of hate. The snake hisses in response and arcs up, ready to spring into action.

"No, not yet," I command with a power I didn't know I had. Anger becomes rage spinning inside of me. Things explode. I'm a nuclear blast and a sucking black hole.

My body jumps at the shrill ring of the school bell. *"What just happened?"* I wonder as I collapse back in my seat, exhausted. I blink hard and look around the room. Kids are gathering their books and bags. Everything looks slightly gray. The grayness enters me and sits heavy on my chest. I feel sick. I'm really losing it.

"Yes, you are losing it," hisses the snake. *"You should be scared of yourself. You don't know what you are capable of."*

My skin prickles. I reach up to brush my hair out of my eyes and feel sweat on my forehead. As I get up from the seat my legs shake. Books clutched to my chest, I stare at the dirty floor as I move to my next class. The warrior I was is gone. My skin continues to crawl and peel away. Fear grips my belly.

What is going on with me?

THE SMOKY QUARTZ

THE BUBBLES COALESCE AND raise me up higher than I've ever been before. I'm one hundred feet tall. I look down at the robot-people shuffling through the mall and imagine squashing them under my feet. I could destroy this entire mall if I wanted to. The idea of this makes me laugh.

The sound of my laugh ricochets off the tile floors. The small insignificant people wandering the mall pause in their conversations to see where the noise is coming from. The darkness in my stomach pulses hotly as I meet their gaze, daring them to say something to the giant I am.

My friend, Ashley, rides my wave of rebellion. We laugh, skipping and running under the florescent lights, leaving open-mouthed stares in our wake. I see the smoky snake ahead of me, slithering in long zig-zagged loops down the tile floor ahead of us, calling me to come forward.

I stop short in front of a crystal shop. Ashley crashes into me from behind. The snake curls around my feet and then moves up to draw a circle around a crystal necklace in the window.

I take in the dark gray color of the pendant that just barely catches the light. This is different than the clear crystal I've had for years. That stone is pure and reflects light. This smoky crystal takes me into the grayness and holds me captive.

I smile as I see the darker hues of gray encased in the crystal, cutting and dividing the smooth grey tone. These ribbons of darkness remind me of my snake. A wave of heat pulses up from my belly into my chest and expands out towards the crystal. I have to have it.

I grab Ashley's hand and enter the store. As I reach out to claim my prize with my other hand, a cold whisper shoots down my spine. I pause, looking over my shoulder. There is nothing there.

"Lauren, are you going to get it?" Ashley asks. The goose bumps leave at the sound of her voice.

"Yes."

As I hold the cool stone my feet start to vibrate. The goose bumps return and I hear a whisper coming from somewhere. I look around again but there is nothing to see.

The title of a book on a nearby bookshelf catches my eye: *The Power of Crystals.* Maybe this is the protection I've been seeking. I drop Ashley's hand and grab the book, my other hand still clutching the crystal. The information about the smoky quartz seems to download into my brain before I even read it:

Smoky quartz is a very protective and grounding stone. It brings physical and psychic protection.

Yes, I need protection.

As a root chakra stone, smoky quartz enhances survival instincts.

Yes, I need to survive.

It is a helpful stone for enhancing and encouraging courage and inner strength.

Yes, I need courage and strength.

Because smoky quartz transforms and removes negative energy, it also protects and cleanses the aura and astral bodies. It can be used effectively for psychic shielding.

Yes, I need a shield.

Soak the crystal in salt water each night to remove the negative energy. This will purify the stone and the wearer.

Yes, I need purification.

I look up from the book and see my snake gliding past the bookshelf, its hiss now sounding like music to me. I briefly bow my head to it in thanks.

I'M NOT ALONE ANYMORE

I'M BEING WATCHED. The pinpricks of stares poke at me. My skin burns. My one safe haven has been compromised. How did this happen? I scan my bedroom with squinty eyes: who is here and how did they get in?

My room looks like it always does: soft peach and green tones, my favorite reading nook, my queen-size, four-poster bed my parents bought for me when I was twelve. All my stuff is where it should be but there is something different. There is someone here.

I stand very still in the corner, pressed in between my closet and my dresser. My breath is locked in my chest. I listen and look, but hear and see nothing. I close my eyes. Is it the whispers of the kids at school? No. Is it the snake? No. Its hiss has become familiar to me, comforting. It's not here. What is it?

More pinpricks poke at me, more heat flushes. A rush of cold air tickles my ear. I grab at my smoky crystal pendant hanging around my neck. I remember the cold whisper I heard the day I bought it at the store. The whisper enters my ears and nose, filling my head with a loud humming noise. Is it the crystal? I whimper as the humming rattles my brain. A rush of nausea rises up from the angry seed.

"You are being watched," the whisper informs me.

"Nowhere is safe," it reminds me.

"What are you going to do now?" it taunts me.

I squeeze my hands against my ears and shut my eyes tight, hoping it will go away. There is a scream in my head. Is that it or me?

My bedroom door opens suddenly. My mom pokes her head inside, "Lauren, are you ready to go?" The humming, pinpricks and heat leave immediately.

"Yes," I mutter breathlessly.

"You okay?" she asks, wrinkling her forehead.

I force a small smile as I look at her and say, "Fine. I was just looking for my leg warmers. I have them now."

She looks at me a moment longer and then turns and walks away, leaving my bedroom door open. I follow after her. Maybe if I'm not alone I'll be okay. Maybe if I'm around others this new scary thing will leave me alone.

I pause in the doorway and look around my room one more time. It looks the same: beautiful, peaceful, normal. But now I know better. Nowhere is safe.

The smoky quartz isn't protecting me, in fact it seems to be tied to the cold whisper somehow. I touch the stone again wondering if I should take it off. I slide my fingers up the chain, unclasp it, and quickly put the necklace on top of my dresser.

What will protect me now?

SAVANNAH

CLIP CLOP CLIP CLOP...

The horses' hooves on the cobblestone street make a sweet kind of music. Their rhythm combined with the gentle sway of the horse-drawn carriage is soothing. The pulsing in my stomach, the dark angry seed and my slithering snake are all gone. Did they know I needed a break? Or now that we're in Georgia, are we too far from home for them to find me?

I breathe deeply and lean back into the red cushions in the carriage, gazing up at the dark sky. This vacation to Savannah is just what I needed. Spring break always feels like freedom—freedom from schoolwork and tests. This year it is also freedom from the bullies at school, the whooshing of the whispers, the hunting ground that has become my daily life. I forgot how easy life can be.

The humidity presses comfortably on me and the warm air tickles my nose. A bubble starts to form in my belly. It feels like an old friend who is as excited to visit as I am to see it again after so long apart. I giggle. The sound is foreign to me: it's been so long since I've laughed.

Mom meets my eye from across the carriage and smiles at my laugh. Dad reaches for her hand as he joins in her smile. Drew points to the old cemetery of Savannah and tells our favorite family cemetery joke.

"Lauren, how many people do you think are dead in there?" he smiles mischievously.

"Ah, all of them?" I respond, smiling.

The guide driving the carriage tells us more stories about hauntings and ghost sightings. I look around eagerly wanting to see something, but I don't.

After our midnight ghost tour we head back to the hotel. While everybody else gets ready for bed I stand outside on our terrace. It's quiet out here. I breathe in the humidity. As the wind picks up I turn towards it, opening up and allowing it to enter me. I breathe in deeply as it sweeps through me. I breathe out, smiling.

I become aware of whispers. They aren't audible words; they're more like invitational tugs on my attention. Just like at the railroad tracks, I begin to feel led by the wind and the whispers. This energy is different though. At the railroad tracks there was only one whisper, this feels like a group of wind whisperers pulling at me.

What do they want me to see? The tug is coming from the left. Isn't the old cemetery over there? They pull at me with more strength than I felt at the tracks. The hotel and gardens begin to fade away. All I see is a path ahead of me like a tunnel through the night.

I take a few steps towards the front lawn. But then the familiar tug of my family inside the hotel room makes me pause. *"What are you thinking?"* I hear a voice inside. *"You can't go wandering off into a strange city in the middle of the night."*

I jerk back from the pull of the whispers and the tunnel disappears. I shake my arms and turn around. The voice is right. That would be crazy to go wandering into the night following the tug of these . . . of these . . . what are they even? What was that?

As I walk through the door into the hotel room the whispers melt away. But now I want to know. . . what is the wind trying to tell me? What are these whispers?

DANCING WITH KNIVES

I GAZE INTO MY eyes in the full-length mirror in my parents' bedroom. The bright red lipstick I've put on makes my eyes pop.

They are pulsing and shining. They remind me of the flashing lights of a disco ball, only with shades of blue, gray and green.

My mouth turns upwards but it's just my reflection smiling. I do not feel this smiling energy inside of me as the performance begins. I'm pulsing, vibrating, popping, just like my eyes.

I look down at the outfit I'm wearing, specially chosen for my dance. The bright yellow of the tulle makes my skin glow. The white blouse has ruffles and with the green vest pressed up tightly beneath my chest, I actually look like I have breasts. I touch the yellow cord that crisscrosses down my belly, ending with a bow at my waist.

I wore this same outfit for a Bavarian folk dance a few years ago. As I gaze at myself in the mirror I don't feel like that girl. I don't look like her either. *Who is this woman before me?*

I breathe in sharply. A rush of heat flows from my belly up to my face. I straighten my spine like a good ballerina and shift sideways just a little bit so I can see more of my shape: the curve of my chest expanding with my breath, the arch of my back, the roundness of my bottom. Another breath moves through me causing my breasts to rise. I look like the women I've seen in movies: sexy, desirable temptresses.

My yellow skirt flairs out at my tiny waist and ends with a white ruffle many inches above my knees. The heat in my belly flows down into my legs. I stretch my left leg out high to the side and point my toes. I watch my calf muscle change from a tight ball to a long slender baton as I alternate between pointing and flexing my toes.

I am a dancer with lines and curves. All my training has sculpted me into a piece of art. The low cut of my blouse shows off my collarbones, as though they are on display. They are like exquisite carvings, so perfect and symmetrical.

I see the pulsing vein on the left side of my neck. I feel the blood moving through it, pushing its way through my body. That's when I allow myself to glance over and see the silver knife resting against my right thigh. My heart quickens at the sight of it. Another wave of heat rushes over me, filling my body.

I lift my right arm slowly and the large butcher knife that I confiscated from the kitchen rises into the air. I am no longer a ballet dancer dancing the safe steps of a Bavarian folk dance. I am a sword dancer. My body twirls and arcs, all the while I watch my reflection.

The knife my partner.

I slide the flat side along my ruffle-covered chest, then angle it so the sharp edge rides over my arm, making the hairs stand up on end . . . in delight? In protest?

I raise both of my arms into the air. My right hand holds the handle of the knife tightly, while the silver point slashes the space above me as though ripping a hole in the sky. My left hand, fingers poised and pressed backwards, receives the weight of the world falling through that hole in the soft white skin of my palm. My arms tense and tingle, my biceps and triceps flexing and softening, flexing and softening.

I glance over at the red numbers of the digital clock on my parents' bedside table. It's 3:40.

The knife my weapon.

I bring the knife to the pulsing vein in my neck and slide it down my arm. I imagine slashing my wrists and watching the blood run down my bare skin, splashing the yellow tulle of my dress. I imagine an invisible audience watching me, unable to stop me from cutting my body, one long slice after another. Blood pours down my outfit and pools at my feet. My beautiful and perfected form destroyed in front of their eyes.

I glance over at the red numbers again. It's 3:45.

The knife my megaphone.

"Look at what you are doing," I yell silently to my imaginary audience. *"Look at the beauty of life you are destroying."* There is so much beauty in this world and nobody is paying attention. They are so busy judging and condemning. They need a wakeup call. Will this get their attention?

Will my ritual sacrifice wake them up to see all the death and destruction they are causing? If not this, then what?

I glance over at the red numbers again. It's 3:50. Ten minutes before Mom comes home from work.

I rise up on my toes in one last grand gesture. I raise my hands over my head with the wooden handle of the knife clutched between them. I am tall, lean, powerful and omnipotent. A flicker of a whisper runs through my head, *"God help me. God, what is wrong with me? God notice me."* And then it is gone.

I lower from standing on pointe and pause, flat footed, taking one last look at my reflection in the mirror. The imagined blood pooled at my feet fades; the disco balls of my eyes still flash and pulse.

Nine minutes later when my mom walks in the house, my lipstick is wiped off, I'm wearing denim shorts and a pink t-shirt, my Bavarian outfit is hanging in my closet and the knife has been returned to the kitchen drawer where it belongs.

"Hi Mom," I call out from where I sit on the living room sofa. And the sword dancer rests until it is time to dance again tomorrow.

4

The Diagnosis

THE FINAL STRAW

THE TEASING AND MOCKERY in school carry over to my one safe haven outside of the family circle—the one place I have felt the most expressive and like me—the dance studio.

I hear snickers constantly. My head snaps up quickly to take in an exchange between the culprits. I feel assaulted. *"It's about me, I know it,"* screams in my mind. I quickly assess all the movements I've just done, looking for what I've done wrong. I try to make myself small and invisible but it's hard to do in a room full of mirrors.

I can't stand it anymore. The crystal isn't protecting me. The knife dancing is my only solace but ten minutes a day isn't enough. I need something else. I begin to wonder about the ibuprofen I carry in my dance bag. I use it to take away any physical pain, just like the other girls in my class do. Will the pills take away the pain I feel when people talk about me?

I decide to try an experiment. After the next round of snickers at the dance studio I calmly take 2 pills and wash them down with the metallic water from the fountain in the front lobby of the studio. Just like the ibuprofen relaxes my muscles after dancing all day, the pills begin to relax my mind, too.

Over the next few days I start taking pills every time I hear laughter or whispers. The pills help me feel a little bit better for about an hour. Is this a sign from God? Does He want me to take more pills? The grayness, the pain, the torment and meanness are too much. I turn back to Him as a final plea. I need Him to help me now.

Every time I feel the tug of someone talking about me I see it as a sign from God: time to take another pill. I want Him to know I'm listening. Maybe then He will start listening to me. My pill intake continues to increase while waiting for a response from Him. Several more days pass and nothing changes. *"Make it stop, God,"* I beg, *"Everything is too loud, too much. Make it stop."*

God isn't listening to me, *again*. Am I truly that bad?

I WANT OUT

I SIT ON THE floor alone in my room, my legs curled into my chest. I rock side to side and watch the sky change from vivid reds and pinks to purple and then finally, blackness.

The color has all faded, just like it has in me.

I am ashes, all ashes. The fire that burned me up must have done the same to the angry seed in my belly. I can't feel it anymore. My snake sits next to me. It's now a diffuse mess of gray, too.

As darkness covers the sky my snake covers me. The dull grayness blankets me from all sides. What's left to do?

FAREWELL LETTER

MAYBE I AM SUPPOSED to die. Maybe dying is my way out of this mess. I retreat to the basement to compose my farewell letter.

I listen to record after record to find the right song to dedicate to each person in my life. I write a paragraph to each person, instructing them to listen to their chosen song to know how I feel about them. Perhaps this way we can still connect with each other even after I'm gone.

My letter offers assurance to my family that they will be okay, they have each other, they have my brother. My friends have one another. I am not really needed. This is really for the best: they'll see this in time.

In the ten long rambling pages I write I call out to everyone to snap out of their slumber and see the beauty around them. I am comforted as I imagine that in my death I can wake them up. God gives me a sense of peace as He is in this plan with me.

When my letter is complete I lay it next to my pillow. I swallow my largest dose of ibuprofen yet. I chase ten pills with water as I pray to God to take me in the night. I let him know I'm ready to carry out our plan.

I wake up groggy and more confused than ever that I'm still alive. I tuck my suicide note in my desk and drag myself forward in my day, going through the motions. All the while feeling my suicide letter awaiting my return.

"I'll try again tonight," spins on an endless loop in my mind.

DISCOVERY

IT'S A GRAY, FLAT DAY. The thick clouds feel oppressive. It's as though the suffocating dullness inside of me is leaking out of my pores and into the world around me.

I drag my tired body home from the school bus stop. My legs feel like they've been filled with concrete. The thought, *"I'll try again tonight,"* circles through my mind like a runner on a track.

Around and around and around. This promise and threat give me a little glimmer of something... hope? Relief? Resignation?

I round the corner of our cul-de-sac and as I look up I see Dad's car in the driveway. He usually isn't home this early. I shrug my shoulders and keep moving forward, putting one concrete leg forward after the other.

I enter into our house through the garage into the laundry room and close the door behind me. The silence enters me like a knife, penetrating the fog I'm in. Something is off. I quickly turn the corner into the kitchen. Both of my parents are sitting at the table. They look up at me with red puffy eyes.

On no: the suffocating sadness has spread to them too. They had tried so hard to keep that from happening. Our house has never felt so sad. The air around us is filled with a heavy helplessness.

Without a word I drop into my usual spot at the table in between them both. My backpack is still on and squishes me close to the table. They reach out for me, Mom holding my right hand, Dad holding my left.

"I found your letter," Mom says. I smile and start to giggle. I know it is inappropriate but I can't help it, a bubble escapes before I have a chance to squelch it.

"Don't. Please don't smile now." Mom says, her voice choked with a sob. I take a breath and shove my giggle down and tuck my lips in.

Mom shares with me what happened, how my teacher called her at work to express her concern about me. Ms. W. could tell I had forged Mom's signature on a note from school that was supposed to inform my parents I had recently gotten a D in Math. This was so unlike me that Mom left work and came home. She told me she had a feeling she needed to search my room, which she did, finding my note in my little desk. That's when she called Dad to come home.

As she talks she and Dad stroke my hands. My body tightens. The usual gentleness of their touch is gone. Instead there's a slight pulling of skin on skin. It agitates me.

I take a deep breath and focus all my energy on not pulling my hands away from theirs. Somehow, someway, my hands are like lifelines for them. If they can grasp my hands perhaps they can make sure I'll never leave them.

I'm not sure what to say or how to justify the letter. I just sit between Mom and Dad watching them stroke my hands. Mom tells me she called Rosemary, the pastor's wife, who is also a clinical psychologist. She is expecting us.

We leave almost immediately to see Rosemary at their house. We drive in silence. Dad is behind the wheel holding my mom's left hand as she wipes tears from her eyes with her right hand. I stare out the window lost for words. What's going to happen now?

Rosemary greets us at the door, holding her 3-week-old newborn in her arms. He's fussy and squirms, as though responding to my own discomfort.

As we walk into the house her toddler peeks around the corner smiling at me. I wiggle my fingers at her to say hello and crouch down to invite her into a hug. She giggles as she tightly grabs my neck. Her joyful bubbles start to spread to me through our hug but I don't let them get far.

The heavy seriousness among the adults needs to be respected. After giggling at the table with my parents I'm trying to match the mood better. I release the little one from our hug after just a moment so her joy can't get to me.

I stand quietly and watch my parents put the toddler and newborn in a stroller. They are going for a walk while Rosemary and I talk. With their attention off me for a moment I have a chance to catch my breath. I shift back and forth, trying to loosen the tightness I feel.

After they leave Rosemary turns to me and smiles, "Let's go sit in my office and talk." I've always liked Rosemary. She is warm and sweet and comforting. The twinkle that I usually see in her eyes when she laughs isn't there today.

She leads me down the steep staircase into the darker basement. Late afternoon light comes through the windows that give me a glimpse of their backyard. Rosemary and I sit on the couch, facing each other. I glance into her eyes then look away, out at the trees. Seeing the trees and green grass relaxes me a little bit.

She knows just what to ask and when to be quiet. The floodgates open. I talk with her for over two hours, surprised at how fast the words pour out of me describing the confusion, pain, doubt, sadness and other turbulent emotions I have been struggling with.

She doesn't judge me. She doesn't accuse me of being crazy. I shake with relief as I finally let myself cry and my body release. My secret is no longer locked up inside of me. Finally, someone is listening. Finally, I'm speaking.

At the end of our session she goes upstairs to invite my parents, who have returned from their walk with the little ones, to sit with us. Rosemary pulls out a sheet of paper from her desk and asks me to read it. It's a suicide contract, she explains. She asks me if I'm willing to sign it, thereby agreeing to not kill myself.

I sign it, knowing that I don't want to die. I never really did. I just want all the noise and chaos around me to stop. I want to be normal. I want to be able to be around people without feeling like I have to cover my ears, squeeze my eyes shut and ball up into a fetal position. I just want the world to be quiet and I didn't know how to make that happen other than silencing myself forever.

THE TURNING POINT

IT HAS BEEN TWO days since my letter was discovered. Two days since my talk with Rosemary. The relief I felt in talking with Rosemary didn't last long. Something else took its place: the truth that there is something seriously wrong with me.

Over the next few days, that fact gets driven deeper into me like a nail into a piece of wood as I talk with my brother and my best friend. I tell them about my depression, the pills and wanting to die. Just the little bit I share seems like too much.

My brother cries. My best friend, whose uncle killed himself when she was young, gets so angry with me that she leaves our house without talking to me. The lines in my parents' foreheads grow deeper during these two days, too.

Already the kitchen knives are locked away, the pills have been thrown out and the window I used to climb out to sit on the roof has been locked. It is clear: I am not to be trusted. We walk on eggshells. No more teasing and easy laughter. Instead the house becomes quiet and somber as though someone has died.

I move through the house with my shoulders slumped and my gaze down. No more perfect ballet posture. I wish I could just disappear. I wish everything could return to normal. My wish is not to be granted.

My parents make an appointment at a fancy clinic so we can get some answers and solutions. That appointment isn't for a week. Rosemary recommends they take me to see a psychiatrist as soon as possible, "Just in case." So three days after my visit with Rosemary, my mom takes me to see my first-ever shrink. She isn't going to diagnose me; she will determine just how suicidal I am.

My belly twists and churns as we drive along the busy 4-lane highway. What will this doctor be like? What questions will she ask? What will she say about me? Will her answers drive the nail in deeper?

My mom slows the car down and turns into a driveway next to a pretty yellow building. It looks more like a country house than a shrink's office building. The rolling hills and maple trees surrounding it greet me. Spring has shifted into early summer and the deep green of the Virginia foliage is on display. The lushness of the new growth feels like a cushion I can relax into. I sigh. The clench in my stomach softens.

As I step out of the car, the sound of the traffic from the highway disrupts my country picture of peace. The noise rips through me. I freeze. Mom takes my hand and leads me inside.

The doctor is a mousy lady with badly dyed hair. She greets us at the door and invites us in to her office. This time Mom comes with me and sits at my side as I answer the doctor's questions.

This meeting feels so different than the one I had with Rosemary. I could feel Rosemary's care in the questions she asked and the way she listened to me. This doctor doesn't seem interested in me at all. She definitely doesn't care about me. Why should she? I'm just a puzzle that she's trying to solve.

"Do you still want to die?"

Did I ever? I don't have an answer. My mother is holding my hand tightly and I can hear her pleading in her head. *"No you don't want to die. No you don't want to leave."*

"No, I don't want to die anymore," I reply in a quiet voice.

"Good." The mouse says. "Then you won't mind signing this."

It's another suicide contract stating I won't kill myself. What is it with these contracts? Everyone seems to think it is such a big deal. Like someone signing it will ensure they will be around forever. Like this will win back their trust. I sigh and sign my second contract stating I won't try to take my own life. My mother and the mouse look pleased.

"You'll have many appointments in the near future to find a diagnosis. We will check everything out to make sure we know what is wrong and what needs to be fixed. In the meantime I'm prescribing a sedative that you can take if things get to be too much."

My mother bristles at the word "sedative." I bristle at the words "wrong" and "fixed." We both sit with our breath sucked in, spines straight and guards up. What have I gotten myself into? Mom takes the prescription and tucks it calmly into her purse. Her eyes meet mine and I can read her mind, *"No way are we using this."*

I lean back into the couch. I'm exhausted. My attention drifts and I feel like I could float away. And then, as my mom continues talking with the doctor, something in her voice pulls my attention back into the room. She's concerned about medicating me before there is a diagnosis. She also asks about what they can do for me before we go to the fancy clinic and if there are any other tests we should do.

Their conversation fades away as the words "wrong" and "fixed" circle around in my head. My mom's worry ripples through me like little shock waves. I can't seem to do anything right. Not saying anything to anyone about what was going on with me didn't work. Now talking about what I'm going through seems to cause pain. "Wrong, fixed, wrong, fixed," keeps echoing through my head. The words get louder and faster.

The gray cloud of the snake begins to stir. It's been lying like a heavy blanket on me since the other night. Now it swirls around me and coils in its loopy form at my feet. The snake's familiar hiss makes the words slam around my head now and my head starts to ache.

"You are hurting people. You're dangerous," chides the snake.

I stiffen. I look over at my mom and the mouse. They are still talking. They obviously don't see the snake. Am I just imagining the snake? Is this a delusion? Maybe I've been making everything up.

"Yes, you are delusional. You have been making it up. You're a liar," bites the snake.

Now I'm really confused. If the snake is a delusion, something is seriously wrong with me. And if I'm not making it up . . . well something is still seriously wrong. I can't tell what is real and what isn't. I can't trust myself.

"No you can't," the snake hisses as it rubs against my legs like my cat does.

Maybe I just need to be normal. Maybe they—the doctors we are going to see at the big clinic—can help me be normal. Maybe they'll have medications that can make me better.

"I can help you," the snake whispers seductively.

"How?"

"I can make you blend in. You're too loud, too noticeable. You are in danger with what you say. I can help you control that."

"How?" I ask again

"It's easy. Just be what others want you to be. You'll be safe. You'll be normal."

It can be easy? I can be safe? There is a way out of this? I feel a shiver in my chest.

In that moment the snake strikes. It uncoils and in an instant its smoky body disappears up my legs. It travels through my pelvis and my belly where the angry seed used to live. It moves along my spine and slithers into my brain.

I look through a gray haze and see my mom and the mouse. They're still talking and although I can't make out their words, I keep my eyes on them. I strain to hear their words. I begin to look for the cues for how to act.

THE "OH" MOMENT

ANOTHER QUIET RIDE IN the car. My parents and I have taken so many trips lately to different doctors: one doctor for my body, one doctor for my brain, one doctor for this, one doctor for that.

The mouse had recommended getting my other testing done before I went to the big clinic, to make sure something else wasn't wrong with me. I've seen my pediatrician, I've had blood work, I've had educational testing... It's been a busy two weeks. My head is blurry from meeting so many people and from explaining myself over and over again like reciting lines in a boring play.

Today is different though. I'm going with my parents to one place where we'll spend the entire day meeting with multiple doctors. Today I am to be diagnosed.

We park the car and walk together towards the three-story brick building, me in between my mom and dad. I look up at my mom and she squeezes my hand. I look over to my dad and he smiles, one of his soft sad smiles I've seen more of these past two weeks.

We enter the building and I hit up against an invisible wall. I feel like I'm walking through a thick cloud. My eyes water and everything looks a little blurry. This is so different from the feeling of the wind on my skin or the pressure before a thunderstorm. This cloud is oppressive. I need to push through it to take a seat in the waiting room.

My chest tightens. It's getting hard to breathe. My skin seems to pull tighter to my bones, squishing all the air out. I swallow and hear the sound of this loud in my ears: "glump." There are a dozen other people around us; other parents with their children, from toddlers to teens. The air is filled with static. I keep my eyes down and stay close to my mom's side.

We don't have to wait long before a stern-looking nurse calls my name. I'm led away from my parents down the hallway. The farther away we walk from them, the tighter my throat gets. It's really hard to breathe now.

The nurse leads me through a maze of hallways before arriving at a door with a nameplate on it. I don't even register the letters on the gold plate as a name. I look up at the nurse as she opens the door. Without even looking at me, she says, "Go on in and have a seat. The doctor will be with you in a moment."

I enter the small office and the door shuts quietly behind me. It's a small room with two chairs, a table and a mirror. A moment later the doctor enters the room. He's wearing a suit and tie. "Hello," he says as he sits down across from me. He takes out some cards from the case he's holding.

He tells me we're going to play a kind of game: he'll show me cards with images on them and I'm to say the first thing that comes to mind. I've heard about these kinds of tests. It's what's used to see if you're crazy.

He shows me the first card. I'm slow to respond. These abstract images of black blobs on white cards confuse me. They could be anything. What does the doctor want me to say? Is there one correct answer?

"A footprint," I say, "A footprint made by someone who has stepped in blood because of all the splatters."

The doctor nods and then holds up the next ink blot card. His stiff face reminds me of the "poker face" my dad puts on when we play cards so I can't guess what's in his hand. Should I put on my poker face, too?

We continue on this way, card after card. What are my answers telling the doctor? I know he's looking for the kink in my wiring so he can figure out the problem. If I can give the doctor what he is looking for then maybe, just maybe, I'll be okay.

So I sit in the chair in the little office, test after test, answering his questions like it's an exam at school. I look at his tie when I respond with my soft voice. Every answer I give seems to open a door inside me that the doctor walks through. He's searching and searching. I shove my hands under my thighs and press my legs down on them, mashing them into the wooden chair. I want to give him what he's looking for, but I don't know what it is or where it is.

After a few hours and more strange tests, I'm given a snack and then ushered to another room. This room has big puffy black leather chairs and photographs on the wall of plants and a waterfall. I say hello to the plant in the pictures and breathe the deepest breath I've had all day. I sink down into one of the chairs and it wraps itself around me. I imagine it's my mom, giving me a hug.

A new doctor comes in with a mustache and warm brown eyes. He actually smiles at me and I melt a little bit into the chair. No poker face with this man. We begin a different kind of testing with question after question. No ink blots to decipher.

This kind of test is easier for me to figure out. Just like the wind nudged and whispered to me, giving me a sense of direction, I feel the same kind of nudging with the doctor's questions. I tune in for his wind whisper and answer the questions. Where will this take us? Like Alice in Wonderland falling down the tunnel . . . if I open this door, what will it lead to?

"Do you have moments when you're sad?" he asks.

A whisper grabs my attention and pulls me to a memory of last summer. I can tell he wants details and he asked about sadness. And I like him. How can I give him what he wants?

As I share the scene from the beach that day, I feel an invisible thread weaving us together: me and the doctor, me and the little blond-haired girl . . .

I'm sitting on my favorite striped beach towel staring at the ocean. I am tired. I wish a storm cloud would come—it would match my mood better. I hear high-pitched laughter and see a little girl running across the beach. She reminds me of how I used to feel: happy. I keep my eyes on her, hoping the bubbles of happiness she's riding will lift me up, too. But they don't. Instead, I feel even sadder. Will I ever be happy again?

As I describe this memory to the doctor I am absorbed in the sadness I felt that day. He's listening to me like he really cares, like he really wants to help me. I look at him through my watery eyes: has he gotten caught up in my sadness? Are those tears too?

He clears his throat and leans back in his chair, straightening his already straight tie. I sit back in my chair too, exhausted. What has my story told him? Can he fix me now?

He stands up and says he'll be right back. He returns a few moments later with my parents. When they see me, they both turn their lips up in an attempt at a smile and take a seat next to me across from the doctor.

Now it's their turn to answer questions. "Do you have a family history of depression?"

Mom, who is usually friendly and open, pauses before responding. She looks back and forth between the doctor, me, Dad and the door as though she is unsure if it's okay to share what she's about to say.

In a stiff, slow voice she shares how her own mother tried to kill herself. How she went to a hospital and was committed. Dad sits quietly at her side, his hand on her back, looking over at me occasionally. I can hear him sending a message to me, "It'll be okay."

Mom is quick to say she doesn't think Grandma really wanted to die. She just wanted to get attention from Grandpa. She also shares how my grandma only stayed at the hospital for a couple of days and during that time she made tea for the

other patients and led the arts and crafts projects. It was clear
she wasn't depressed or suicidal and was released after only a
day or two.

"Anyone else?" the doctor asks.

Mom takes a big breath and then in one big exhale says,
"My sister is bipolar."

"Oh."

The doctor turns his head and looks at me. I can see the
puzzle pieces coming together in his mind. He knew about the
suicide attempt and the knife dancing and the sadness. Now he
just needs more information to complete the picture.

His "Oh" response feels like a stake in the ground; like he
now knows where he is going and it's my job to follow him. I see a
tunnel open up before us and I follow his lead. He asks me some
more questions.

"Do you have trouble sleeping?"

Where are we going? "Yes."

"Do you have uncontrollable energy?"

We continue to move down the tunnel. "Yes."

"Do you get really happy sometimes?"

Duh—of course. "Yes."

"Do you feel really happy and then get sad?"

Have you been listening to anything I have said? "Yes."

"Do you swing from one to the other?"

Deeper we go down the tunnel. I'm being pulled to follow.
"Yes."

I don't feel like I am answering as me. His desire to go down
this tunnel pulls at me. I'm curious as to where we will go. So
I keep agreeing with him. Saying no at this point doesn't seem
right. Maybe there is something at the end of the tunnel that will
help me.

The doctor makes some notes on his clipboard and then looks up at my parents. Oh good, he's figured it out. Now we'll know. Now they can fix me.

"She has bipolar."

With that one word my parents come undone. I can feel their worlds crumbling. It's like a thousand bees escape and are buzzing around us all. What does this mean? My parents don't seem relieved at this answer. My curiosity about the tunnel seems to have gotten me into trouble. Something is very wrong.

The doctor talks about rapid cycling and a need for medications: mood stabilizers, anti-depressants, anti-psychotics . . . My aunt's face comes to mind. The one with bipolar. She has a very rocky life. Did I go down the wrong rabbit hole?

Then I hear the doctor talk about another option. "We can commit her and watch her twenty-four hours a day. We can adjust the medicine and see their effects sooner. This is the quicker track to stabilizing her."

Yes, I think. This is the way to go. The quicker track. Stabilize me.

"Yes," I say.

My parents look over at me. Their eyes open even wider. *"Noooooo,"* I hear the unspoken cry in my mother as she starts to shake.

I feel tricked. I thought I was doing the right thing by following the doctor down this tunnel. But now everything feels wrong. I don't like seeing my mom cry. I don't want to see that look in their eyes anymore. I want to leave.

A buzzing sound fills my head. I drift up and away from my body, floating near the ceiling, looking down at my body, which remains sitting at the table next to my parents. The doctor continues to talk yet all I hear is "Check in on Monday."

I watch from the ceiling as my parents get up from the table and help me to my feet. I feel like one of those marionettes that move with someone else's hands on the controls.

FLOATING

I FLOAT THROUGH THE next couple of days as we prepare for my big trip on Monday to the mental hospital. I watch my body from above as it operates all on its own. After all the intensity I've felt with the highs and lows, this new experience of nothingness is such a relief. Why didn't I choose this before?

I'm pleased with my new trick. I discover I no longer feel what my parents are feeling. But I can tell they are sad. They try to hide it but they can't. Their eyes are red-rimmed and puffy. Worry lines burrow into their forehead and take up residence.

Occasionally I stop floating to try and feel them again but when I do my body screams. Their sadness is so heavy it's like an elephant sitting on my chest. My faces burns, my eyes sting and I can't breathe. So I float out further where their sadness can't touch me.

I like the fuzzy nothingness when I float. I see everything through a gauze-like film. It's like watching an old movie where the picture is grainy and everything moves really slowly; a movie where I get swept away in the movement of the story and don't pay attention to the details.

My upcoming trip to the mental hospital takes on the energy of a vacation. Small bubbles lift me up further. I'm excited by the idea of a retreat. Something new and different: this is exactly what I need. I even get to go shopping in preparation.

Mom takes me to the store to buy new make-up. I'm allowed to get anything I want with one caveat—it has to be in a plastic tube. For some reason they don't allow glass where I'm going. After we get new eye shadow and foundation we search for an electric razor. I'm not allowed to take my regular razor with me because of the blade.

Mom has a list from the doctors with rules like this. Something about the risk of cutting. I don't know what cutting is and I don't care to. As she reads the list to me I barely listen. She's in the grainy movie again; I focus on the shopping.

Back at the house I discover Dad has laid out his nice suitcase on my bed for me to use. This is the one he uses for his business trips. Now I'm the one who gets to go on an adventure.

I stand in front of my closet for a while, unsure of what to pack. Finally I decide to pack my best outfits to make a good impression. I also pack my ballet clothes, shoes and my favorite music to dance to while I'm there. How else will I be spending my time?

On Sunday morning we go to church as usual. After the service, everyone mills about, socializing in the atrium. The mass of people buzz like a hive of bees. The static becomes intolerable. My head hurts.

Some of mom's friends look at me with odd expressions on their faces. A mixture of, what is that? I can't quite feel it anymore. Concern? Pity? Each look sends an electric shock through my body.

When they talk to me I feel a tug, like they're trying to keep me close. I can't float as easily. I leave the cluster of people and stand on the edge, close to the large glass doors. This way I can keep floating out above everyone, separate from the conversations and concern. The static starts to die down as I float further away.

Something pulls me to look back and I see my mom sniffling. Her three best friends stand close to her. One woman hands her a tissue and the other two rub her back. It's too heavy to watch. I turn back to the window and float away into the trees.

DRIVE TO THE MENTAL HOSPITAL

MONDAY MORNING COMES. I get dressed like any other day. I put on my make-up using the old illicit glass containers since my new stuff is already packed. I put on a dress—one I usually reserve for church or opening days of our theater productions at school.

Dad takes the day off from work again. My parents stare at me while I eat breakfast. They fidget and don't say anything and that makes me fidget. I eat quickly to escape their staring.

We head off in the car. I sit in the back seat gazing out the window. I float up through the puffy white clouds past the bright green new growth on the spring trees. It's my favorite time of year.

After about twenty minutes we pull off the highway and enter the city. It becomes harder to stay up in the sky, floating. The congested roadways and additional people tug at me. It's as though the volume gets turned up again and the sound pulls me back.

I land back in my body as though someone has shoved me into a bucket of ice. Ouch! I gasp out loud at the shock of it. In that instant the reality of where we are going hits me. We are going to a Mental Hospital. This is not a vacation. This is not an adventure I want.

"No!" I scream. "No, I don't want to go there!"

My parents are surprised at my sudden outburst. Dad slows the car to regain control and Mom leans back to take my hand. I continue to scream "No" as my body shakes with sobs. All this time my body was trying to get my attention but I was floating away as far as I could go.

My parents look at each other and I see my mom shake her head, "No" at my dad. He turns the car around even before we hit the next traffic light.

"It's okay Lauren. We won't go if you don't want to," Mom whispers to me softly. I'm surprised I can hear her over my crying.

The mood in the car does a complete 180 degrees like the car just did. My entire body sighs. My sobs quiet and I allow myself to breathe. I make an effort to not float away. I look at my parents with clearer vision—the fuzz has lifted.

Mom calls the hospital on the car phone and cancels my reservation while Dad drives us to a nearby restaurant for lunch. We are all quiet as we sit at the big oak table on the balcony. I enjoy being back in my body and the taste of my favorite sandwich. Today this turkey club tastes like freedom.

5

Being Committed: To Bipolar

REATTACHMENT OF MY UMBILICAL CORD

RATHER THAN BEING COMMITTED at the Mental Hospital, I become committed at home. It becomes the family joke; the kind of joke that lacks any laughter: "Lauren's umbilical cord is reattached."

Mom is now the one with my marionette controls in her hands. She goes to the school board and rallies on my behalf. She gets me released from the last two months of my 8th grade year. I no longer take Math and English, Gym or Art. My new "schedule" includes counseling on Tuesdays and Thursdays, medication checks on Wednesdays, long walks in the woods and lots of sitting on the couch with my cat, Thumbelina, in my lap.

One afternoon I get a headache. As I head to the bathroom cabinet for some ibuprofen I feel eyes on me. Wherever I go, those eyes follow me. Mom's always present watching eyes have replaced the whispers from school. I open the cabinet and scan the shelves. There aren't any pills. I head to my bedroom to check my dance bag but remember I emptied that out when they pulled me out of dance class. I lay on my bed, gazing at the ceiling, feeling the thud-thud of my headache. I can feel Mom's eyes on me, even though my door is closed.

I turn over on my side and hug a pillow to my chest. Now the only pills I take are the ones Mom administers to me every day. She counts out the different pills and makes sure I get the right doses at the right time. She drives me to and from my doctor's appointments. She tells me what to do and where to go, when. All I need to do is follow.

A NIGHT AT THE MOVIES

BEFORE MY DIAGNOSIS, my family loved to play together. We had our boys and girls club—me and Mom paired together just as Drew and Dad did. Drew and I were both respective best friends to our same sex parent. This was driven mainly by interest—the boys liked sports, the girls liked art. Times with all of us together were somewhat rare but always fun. Vacations to Disney or to the beach, movies, dinners, walks outside.

After my diagnosis everything changed. Our camaraderie disappeared. The unspoken questions sat like elephants in the room: Do we talk about Lauren's issues all the time? Do we ignore them completely? Is it okay to joke to lighten the mood? Is it okay to laugh? She just tried to kill herself...

In an attempt to find some semblance of "normal" my mom suggests we all go out to see a movie. It's been a week since our drive to the Mental Hospital, a week of my new schedule of no school, meds and counseling. Maybe a movie will help lighten things up.

Sitting between my mom and brother in a dark theater laughing and eating popcorn is the best medicine I've had all week. I can pretend everything is normal again; that I am normal. At least for this night.

As we walk out to the car after the movie I look up at the stars. I feel a familiar sensation of bubbling in my pelvis. I smile and start to open to these old friends of mine. And then I remember what the doctors told me: that this is the craziness. I press my hand against my belly. Perhaps if I press hard enough the bubbles will go away. It's dangerous to play with this energy.

As we drive home my dad tells stupid jokes that have us all laughing again like we did in the theater, like we did before my diagnosis. He shares joke after joke. As our laughter builds the bubbles in my pelvis return. They are so strong now from being pressed down that there is no stopping them. The bubbles rush up and out of me in the form of big belly laughs. Mom, Dad and Drew are so happy to see me happy they keep laughing. It's as though now I'm the one telling jokes with these hiccupy bubble-filled laughs.

And then something shifts. My laughter intensifies and the bubbles and I get out of sync. I feel like I'm in the ocean trying to surf the waves but they're coming too quickly and I'm being pummeled. The waves drop me and turn into big sobs that rip through my body. The tension from these past several weeks slides out of me in tears and gasping wails.

Mom leans over the front seat and pats my leg, making soft soothing sounds. My brother sits closer to me, fidgeting, not sure what to do or how to make this all better. Dad keeps looking in the rearview mirror at me. Although it's not spoken out loud, I can hear their collective voices saying, *"We are here for you, we just don't know what to do for you, and we're freaking out, too."*

By the time we arrive home, we are all quiet. We get out of the car and head into the house, Mom's arm draped around my shoulders. No more pretending anything is normal.

LEARNING MY NEW ROLE

As I WALK TO the library, the memory of my breakdown in the car last night presses down on me like a heavy gray cloud. My out-of-control bubbles have now ruined almost everything; even movie night isn't what it used to be.

Will we ever return to normal? Can we? What is this bipolar thing? Why do my parents look so upset every time I mention the word?

There is something I'm not being told. I'm sure of it. The glances between my parents along with the knowing looks exchanged between the doctors speak more loudly to me than the information they've shared. It's time for me to find out what this diagnosis is really about.

I open the door to the library and am greeted with the familiar and somewhat musty smell of books. The elderly woman at the reference desk shows me where to find what I'm looking for. I'm grateful she doesn't ask me any questions.

I head to the stacks and find a book filled with different psychological diagnoses. As I check the table of contents looking for bipolar, I see the look in my parents' eyes when we received the diagnosis. Their look of doom makes the words fuzzy.

I rub my eyes and blink several times. Now I can focus. I find what I'm looking for on page 132: a list of bipolar symptoms.

- Mood swings
- Cycles of excessive energy and no energy
- Tendency towards promiscuity
- Excessive shopping
- Pressured fast speech
- Irritability
- Impulsivity

The mood swings and cycles of energy levels are true. I tend to flip very easily as I catch different waves and whispers around me. I guess I'm impulsive—how else would you describe the knife dancing and roof climbing?

I look up at the stacks around me. I don't get it. Some of this fits, but a lot of it doesn't. I haven't been on any shopping binges. I'm not sexually promiscuous; I'm actually really shy around boys. I'm not usually irritable . . .

Am I supposed to be all of these things? If I don't have all these symptoms now, will I develop them later? Are they hiding under the surface just waiting to pop up? What if I don't ever have all of these? Does that mean I'm not bipolar?

I sway a bit in my seat. All of my thoughts speed up and slow down at the same time. I feel like I'm falling. If I don't fit in the "bipolar box," where do I fit? How will the doctors know how to fix me?

A shiver runs up my spine at the thought of starting over again at square one: knowing something is wrong but not knowing what it is and how to fix it. Scenes from this past month flash through my head: the doctors, the questions, and every part of me being poked, searched and invaded. No thank you! I close my eyes and check my body for these symptoms. Where are they?

I remember my drama teacher telling me how great acting is more than memorizing lines, "To be believable as a character you must allow your audience to feel you. You can find any emotion inside of you and bring it up during a scene. You become the emotions; you become the character."

Maybe that's what I need to do. Instead of just learning the facts and researching bipolar like I would a school research paper, maybe it's time to pull up these symptoms from inside of me and become them. Just like I did when I became the character of Helena when we did a performance of Midsummer's Night's

Dream earlier this year. I pulled up her passion to be believable.

I got a standing ovation for that performance. So if I play this bipolar role well, will the doctors be able to fix me once and for all? I leave the library feeling lighter. The heavy gray cloud is no longer pressing against me. I'm now armed and ready to see the doctors. I know how to make this new role of mine believable, thanks to my drama training.

Over the next couple of months, in every conversation with doctors, I share with them my script. I not only list the symptoms, I become them. I talk in the pressurized fast speech the book described. I talk about promiscuous thoughts and behaviors. I act irritable. I play my role as "girl with bipolar" very well.

I hope this convinces the doctors that they have the right diagnosis so they can get on with the work of fixing me. But that doesn't happen. One by one the doctors' words pierce me with daggers as they say things like:

- Bipolar is biologically driven. You will need medicine for the rest of your life.
- Bipolar is hereditary. You will pass this onto your children one day.
- Bipolar is triggered by stress.
- Bipolar people are unpredictable and have a hard time achieving a stable life."
- Bipolar people have a hard time holding down a job and handling money.
- The medicine for bipolar is essential: if you miss a dose you could start to cycle.
- The medicine cannot be mixed with alcohol: if you drink you may get sick or die.

- Bipolar is hard to control with medicine: even with the correct dosage you may still have trouble.

Oh no . . . What role did I take on? Is this what they really mean?

Biologically driven = something is inherently wrong with me

Stress triggered = the shoe could drop at any moment

Unpredictable = I'm dangerous and unsafe to be around

Marching orders = I need to find a way to control myself

I've been so focused on fixing this *right now*. But the doctors are not talking just of now; they are talking about the rest of my life! They are talking about f-o-r-e-v-e-r. You mean I may have to play this role forever?

I'm already stressed out, experiencing the world at such a high volume, the only option for silence I know is to take my own life. I'm in middle school. Middle school! How will I handle the rest of my life?

If I can pass this horrible intensity to my kids, if I need medicine to fix my inherently screwed up biology and if a simple stress could send me into a tailspin, then who would choose to be with me? Who will want to marry me? Have kids with me?

How stupid am I to pick this. What a life . . . what a role.

I feel utterly depressed. I thought this was a cold we could treat and fix, once all the symptoms where identified. I thought this was a temporary role—not a lifetime sentence.

Tightness creeps in with every warning by the doctors. I try to shove the symptoms I pulled from within back down again. Anger churns in my belly. I'm reading myself for battle again—but who or what is the real enemy?

IT'S NOT SAFE TO SHARE

I SIT DOWN ON the old paisley couch and the cushions suck me in. I feel the intense gaze of the doctor on me as I twist my hands and shift from side to side. He is perfectly still on his firm leather chair. He doesn't say anything; he just clears his throat to grab my attention.

I meet his eyes and immediately sense his disapproval of my fidgeting. I cross my legs tightly and clasp my hands together. I sit up as straight as possible in the slumping chair and smile shyly at him.

"Tell me again about what you experience when you are outside," He says calmly as his fingers brush his dark mustache. I clear my throat as the sensation of the hairs on his lips somehow tickles my own throat.

He wants me to talk about sensing the earth. I told him this already. He didn't believe me. He said it was a 'manic' episode. Just as he said the wind whispers were 'hallucinations.' And that I had 'paranoia' because I could hear others talking about me all the time. All these new vocabulary words are upsetting. I have researched them but it feels different when the doctors use them to describe me. When they use these words they feel like daggers being thrown at me.

I sigh, "I told you before. It just felt really good. I could feel the earth pulsing under me but then it wasn't under me it was inside of me. The sky touched my head then and came inside too."

My story has been shortened. My voice has been softened. I leave out the details as they have been shared before and weren't believed. When I tell it now it feels like just a report: it has lost the life it had when I was outside.

The doctor sighs also and makes more scribbly notes on his large yellow legal pad. As usual he holds it out of view so I can't see what he is writing.

He writes for a while. "Anything else?"

"I don't know what else to tell you about it," I reply quietly.

"Have you had any more experiences like this lately?" He probes.

I pause and close my eyes, unsure of how much to share . . .

I think of my daily walks. It is the only time I'm left alone. My parents watch me constantly at home. Mom's eyes follow me everywhere. My one treat is to put on my Walkman with a mix tape Drew made me and go explore outside.

I walk down by the lake close to our house following the paved trail. I don't tell my parents that I not only walk along the path where the houses are but I keep going and cross over the tiny bridge that leads to the woods. As I do I shut off the blare of the Walkman that has buffered out the neighborhood noise so I can enjoy the sounds of nature.

The wooden bridge creaks as I walk over the rough wood. I remember my favorite novel, *Bridge to Terabithia*, each time I cross the bridge because just like in the story I find a magical forest on the other side.

As soon as my foot hits the other side of the path I breathe more deeply. The high grass tickles my bare legs as if in greeting. I hear a rustling sound nearby and send out a silent, "Hello," to the unseen creature.

I follow the dirt path through the woods to where it winds down and meets the creek. I step over the large stones along the side of the creek to where my tree is—a weeping willow with branches that touch the earth.

I crawl beneath her branches and sit listening to the soft gurgling of the water as it flows by. I close my eyes and feel the warm kiss of the sun on my cheeks; the breeze lifts my hair.

I open my eyes and look at the doctor across from me. I open my mouth to tell him about my daily walks but no sound comes out. He won't understand. He never does.

I don't want any more new words thrown at me. I don't want him to tell my parents I pass over the bridge into the woods and not be allowed to go walking alone anymore. I don't want my magical forest to be disturbed by this man's opinion.

"No," I reply. "I haven't had any experiences like that."

He smiles finally, pleased that one 'problem' has been solved. "So now tell me again about the presences you feel."

I tell him the same; that I haven't had any more experiences like what I had by the railroad tracks or in Savannah. He continues to look pleased.

I remember how at the first Youth Group Meeting I went to after my diagnosis I blurted out the real reason why I'd been pulled out of school. Some of my friends were shocked. Some of them cried. I was relieved.

But later that night the phone kept ringing. The parents of the kids in the youth group wanted to talk with my parents. While they were concerned about me, they were also upset because their children were upset.

"People don't know what to do in this kind of situation. They are scared," Dad said.

"You just need to be careful about who you share this with," Mom said, "They may not get it."

I get it though. It's not okay to share any of this stuff. No one understands it. No one else needs to know about it.

6

Cocktail Party

MY BODY IS ANGRY

THE COCKTAIL PARTY of medications begins . . .

The doctors start me on lithium and an anti-depressant. The first anti-depressant doesn't work so they try another one while also increasing the lithium. My body begins to do the strangest thing: my once beautiful face is now covered with red acne. These red lumps spread down my once-clear creamy skin to cover my chest, upper arms and back.

My skin becomes angry and continually erupts. It's stretched so tight with all of this swelling that if I turn my head the spiteful cysts explode and leak. I am in a living nightmare. There is no way to hide or be invisible.

As I walk through the hallways at school and sit in class I feel like a carnival act. Like one of those freaky people you pay to see: the elephant man or the fat lady. I would be called the Erupting Volcano Girl and little children would point their fingers at me screaming, wishing they could run away yet cannot because they are riveted to the red boils that erupt and flow.

I do everything I can to conceal them. Although I can't hide them completely, my stage make-up from dance class helps a bit.

So every morning before school I pull out my makeup and like an artist priming her canvas, I get to work.

I read in a beauty magazine that green tones down red. I spread sage green foundation over my once-perfect skin to balance out the redness. With my pointer finger I dab thick green sticky concealer on the angriest boils that threaten to explode. I paint on another layer of beige foundation to blend this all in to match my skin tone.

I decide my best defense is a good offense so I play up my one remaining pretty feature—my green eyes—with green eye liner and thick black mascara. I don't wear any blush or lipstick: I definitely don't need any more redness on my face and don't want anything to distract from my eyes.

I stare at my reflection in the mirror for several moments after I'm done painting my face. More like a mask than a masterpiece, the stage make-up gives me some protection as I head out to school. Even after all my painting and concealing I can still feel people's eyes on me and hear their whispers as they talk about me. Sitting in chemistry class one day I hear a boy behind me say, "I bet if you just touched that girl you would break out all over." His friend laughs.

I sink further into my seat. I quickly glance up at the teacher. Will she say anything? My face gets even redder and warmer as she joins in on the laughter.

Hearing my classmate say this is one thing, but seeing the teacher laugh? Anger spreads through me like white lightning. I can hear the snake hissing at me, telling me to be quiet, to bite my tongue. I fight the urge to lunge at the teacher.

Instead I curl my hands into fists beneath my desk and keep my eyes on my notebook in front of me, pretending to be absorbed in the homework assignment. I can't risk saying anything. I can't risk looking at her with eyes that want to kill her. Then they would call me crazy. Then they would lock me up. So I stuff my anger down as my skin grows redder and redder.

Every touch, treatment or cure seems to irritate the red lumps even more. My mother takes me to see the dermatologist. I desperately want the doctor to help me. Instead, she makes things worse. "It's a shame," she says as she shakes her head, "You're so pretty."

Her pity nauseates me. A combination of sadness and anger spread through me. I want to cry and scream at the same time. Can no one fix this?

To help reduce the swelling and prevent more scarring the dermatologist injects cortisol into every sensitive red cyst. Each pierce of the needle makes me shiver. The cortisol burns and stings as it spreads slowly through the cyst and beyond it. My mom sits in the room with us, watching and wincing at every injection. My eyes water but I don't allow myself to cry.

At our next appointment with the psychiatrist Mom asks if the lithium is causing these red cysts. The doctor says no. I've researched this though. I know he's lying. I know he knows that kids would rather be crazy than be covered with boils. I don't say anything. Instead of lowering the dosage of lithium, he prescribes more medicines for me: a topical antibiotic and acne medicine.

I hate taking the lithium knowing it's what's causing the red boils. What's even worse is that I have to go see the school nurse every day to take the mid-day dose. Leaving class is like a big sign pointing at me saying, "She's not normal!"

The nurse doesn't help any either. She looks at me with her squinty eyes as she hands me a little white cup with the pale yellow pill in it. It looks like a bug ready to choke me. I take the cup from her and swallow the pill with some water. The nurse asks

me to open my mouth afterwards to make sure I'm not hiding
the pill so I can spit it out after I leave her office. Doesn't she
know I'm too much of a good girl to do that?

"Fuck you," I want to hiss at her. The rage bubbling inside
makes my boils pulse with heat. But I shove the rage down, open
my mouth and lift my tongue for her to check. I smile sweetly at
her as I leave.

I return to class, slinking into my seat hoping nobody will
ask me anything. I don't want to invite attention or leave clues
for people to start piecing together. I need to keep my secret safe.
They don't ask but I'm sure they make up stories about why I
have to go see her every day. Whatever stories they make up, they
can't be worse than the truth.

MY BODY: A PRISON

ALL THESE RED BOILS have sucked the moisture out of me.
I now have unquenchable thirst. My tongue is like sandpaper
and scratches away at the roof of my mouth with each movement. Every cell on my tongue—and in my body—cries out for
liquid. I wake up almost every hour in the night to gulp the water
I've left in an ice bucket by my bed and then go pee.

I drink all the time. My belly swishes and swashes as I move.
Solid food scratches my mouth and makes me even thirstier.
I lose my appetite. The curves of my body that I used to enjoy
watching in the mirror: my butt, my small breasts, my calves,
have all changed. I am a stick figure, a skeleton, the walking dead.

In class one day I run my hands through my thick brown hair
and a clump of it falls out in my hand. I hide it as fast as I can
in a ball in my hands and make my way to the trashcan. On my
way back I notice the trail of golden hair I left in my path, like

breadcrumbs guiding me back to my seat. On and around my desk there are small shiny piles of the same golden threads. My seatmates pretend not to notice. At home I notice more hair on the sink and in my brush. When and how did this happen?

It's hard to concentrate and understand what's being said to me. The teachers at school sound like the adults in the Peanuts cartoon, "Whah wha wha wha whah."

I am still aware of the things that aren't spoken. Like someone else's judgment or fear or anger. The thing they aren't saying out loud. These energies enter me and I feel a rush of pain. Then the fog closes around me again, keeping me numb and quiet. I don't tell anyone about this because I don't want them to think I'm crazy. And talking about this feels like too much effort.

I feel like I'm in jail. My body is a prison. The doctors, the medicine, even my parents are the jailers. I want to claw and scratch at everyone and everything but I'm too tired to do so. The weakness and inability to act pisses me off even more. More rage ensues only to get shoved down deeper as it has no way out past the lethargy.

I feel ugly physically and emotionally. I want to be left alone. I hate the world. I want out. Desperately wanting to be okay and normal, I learn to say, "I'm fine," really quickly. But the feelings and fears I stuff down dig at me. I'm irritated with everything.

I snap at Mom and Dad. They are the ones I feel the safest with so my mini-volcanic-like eruptions occur around them. They look at me with sad eyes when they think I don't see them. I feel their worry. It adds to my own.

Everyone pretends this is all okay. They tell me this will make me stronger. They tell me I'm courageous. I want to yell at everyone, "Shut up! Shut up! Shut up!" And I wonder why do I have to go through all this shit? WHY?

I want all this to stop. My body is out of control. The cocktails of drugs have taken over. I never know what's going to be next. I think it's as bad as it can get and then it gets worse.

MY BODY: A PRESSURE COOKER

IT'S TOO MUCH. Everything is too much. The noise of the hallway between classes vibrates like shock waves through my ears and into my head. I have constant headaches.

The clusters of bodies with hardly any space to move between them are suffocating. Intense smells fill my nose. Everyone is too close. There is no space. It's hard to breathe.

I try to be invisible. I cower inside and shrink my body down. I pull away from everyone to protect myself. But it doesn't work. I can still feel what I've been trying so hard not to feel. Why aren't the medicines fixing this?

There is something wrong. I can't put my finger on what it is. It's not tangible which is disorienting. The anxiety is taking up space and squashing my breath. It is clouding my vision and making my ears ring. It has its hand on my heart and it squeezes so tight it brings tears to my eyes.

It's too much. I can't breathe. Something is pushing its way through my body. It is going to explode out in waves of tears. I can't let anyone see this.

I walk faster through the mix of smelly bodies, past the eyes that watch me. As I tunnel through the spaces between bodies I feel like I'm swimming upriver. My face burns; my breath is caught in my chest. I'm going to explode.

I reach the locked door just in time and pull out the large silver key from my pocket. This is one of the perks of being a drama student aid: a free pass into the backstage area.

I walk into the dark empty space, closing the door behind me quickly just as a cry erupts. My chest tears apart as another sob breaks free. My mouth, tired of being clenched in silence, stretches and lets loose more sobs. The empty theater fills with my wailing. With no audience present there is no need to edit.

I walk quickly back and forth in the long narrow area like a panther at the bars in the zoo. I shake with sobs as tears flow down my cheeks.

I sink against the closed door to the ladies' dressing room. The cold metal against my back sends a shiver through me and calms me. The sobs slow down. My breath still catches and comes out in jagged bursts.

I curl my legs up under my chest into a fetal position. The pressure of the hard floor and the support of the door on my back are comforting. I rock side to side as my breath slowly evens out.

The bell chimes overhead alerting me and the other hundreds of students in the hallways that it's time to get to class. I stand up quickly and wipe my eyes on my tee shirt. I don't want to be late to class. I don't want anyone wondering what's wrong.

I take a final look into the darkened theater. I raise my arms up and stretch them one at a time towards the ceiling. I take a deep breath. Time to stuff the sobs down again as I prepare to step back into the spotlight of my life.

"I'm okay. I'll be okay. I can do this," I whisper to myself quietly, my own private cheerleader.

I slip out the door, closing it softly behind me. With my chin down and books tucked under my arms, I walk through the almost empty hallways and head to class.

My Body: A Pincushion

EVERY SIX WEEKS MY MOM drives me to the blood draw place. The doctors require this: they need to make sure my liver isn't failing from all the toxicity in the drugs. I hate the dark and dank smell inside. We wait for a long time in the reception area before they call me in to the office.

When it's finally my turn the nurse sits me in a cold hard plastic chair that hurts my butt. I roll up my sleeve. "Wow! You have great veins!" she says to me every time, like this is the ultimate compliment. "Which one would you like me to draw from?"

Why do they ask me this? It's irritating how stupid they are. "Just pick one."

I don't look away: I never do. I stare at my milky flesh and the bluish thread underneath it. I watch the cold sharp needle poke and invade me. I watch the dark blood pour into the vile. It doesn't hurt. It just feels wrong.

I don't cry or get emotional. I just observe. I can barely feel it through the medication fog anyway. They bandage me up and send me on my way.

I start to notice permanent holes in my arms after a while. Like there is a spot just waiting to be poked.

Losing What I Love the Most

WHEN I STARTED HIGH SCHOOL, I also started up with dance classes again. Dancing was my favorite thing to do, until it started to become a battle.

One of the drugs they give me causes tremors. I shake uncontrollably. I look nervous all the time. I hate how weak I look and feel. Even the simplest of movements becomes difficult as I quiver and quake.

Now I can't even balance on pointe. I have to concentrate so hard on trying not to shake that I become ridged, losing all sense of the grace and harmony I once enjoyed. I start to hate the thing I loved the most.

The doctor gives me an anti-convulsant to help me during performances and auditions. I'm not allowed to take it every day because it could paralyze my facial muscles. *It could paralyze my face.* Just knowing this makes me tremble before I use it. The meds help me get through a few hours without all the trembling but I wonder... is it worth it?

As if this isn't bad enough, I become filled with gas and have explosive diarrhea. It's difficult to hold it in during dance class. I escape to the bathroom, which unfortunately is close to the dance floor. I turn on the fan to muffle the sound. My bowels explode. I spray deodorant from my dance bag in an attempt to cover the intense smell.

I feel proud of my deception. Nobody will be able to smell this. I make my way back to my mark: front and center. That's when I hear a comment about "the big bang".

I want to crawl away. I want to disappear.

MY BODY: OF INTEREST

AS WE WAIT FOR the bus I tuck my chin in my scarf, trying to protect myself from the cold and from the stares. My girlfriends are talking about the soup kitchen we are volunteering at. We're in Toronto on a mission trip with our youth group.

The bus arrives and as I follow my girlfriends to seats in the back I can feel the hot pinprick of someone staring at me from behind. As I sit down I sneak a peek and see an older man with graying hair staring at me with beady eyes and an ugly grin. I shiver and look away.

I had just told my girlfriends how uncomfortable I feel in my skin, how gross I feel. Now they try to soothe me and make me feel better. "It's not so bad," they say. "It'll get better," they assure me while a few of the older girls share words of wisdom on how to heal acne.

I can tell that the man is listening to our conversation. This grosses me out even more and I slouch down in my seat. The man seems to sense my discomfort, but doesn't look away. He keeps on staring at me as though he can get into me with his eyes.

My girlfriends are off on another subject: one of them has a new boyfriend. I stop listening to them and start to float away.

Again and again I am told how beautiful I am despite my acne. At the prom in my sexy red dress Mom helped me pick out, in drama class when leading choreography while prancing around in spandex, in class as I walk by a group of boys, in all the modeling and acting gigs I do after school.

I am used to people looking at me with disgust when they see the boils and the caked make-up trying to cover them. Then their eyes fall to my figure and I can feel heat rise in my pelvis. It feels good and wrong at the same time.

I don't understand how anyone can find me attractive. And not just because of the boils. Can't they see how messed up I am? Can't they sense the anger that wants to claw their eyes out? Can't they sense my desperation at this crazy life I lead?

The bus comes to a sudden stop and I come back from my floating. The man is getting up to leave. He is still staring at me. I try to hide more. As he crosses in front of me he says in a rough voice, "You know what you could try to heal acne? More sex. From the looks of it you'd need a lot."

With that he turns and exits the bus. I feel the tears come and can't stop them. My friends pat my hand and tell me it'll be okay.

But I know it won't be. I'm tired of being invaded. I'm tired of having people stare and say whatever the hell they want to me. I'm tired of no one caring how uncomfortable I am.

I tuck my chin further into my scarf and feel my boils pulsing.

THE CRASH

ANOTHER COLOR IS ADDED to the rainbow of my pharmaceutical cocktail that I swallow three times a day. It's a new medicine that is supposed to help with depression and social anxiety.

The doctors are excited and say, "This is very promising." I'm filled with doubt as I've heard this many times before . . .

I don't feel any effects of it at first. Usually, with the other drugs it's a slow on-set. A fog clouds over me or fatigue creeps in. This drug is different. It introduces itself to me with no warning one morning while driving to school.

After spending the past three years tied to my mother, the independence of driving is intoxicating. When I am driving I am the queen of my own domain. I choose which roads I turn on and where I go. I'm more alert than any place else when I'm behind the wheel.

This morning is different though. As I drive along the familiar road to school, the fog I live in pools together in my eyes. One minute I see the houses and maple trees lining the road and the next minute I can't see anything.

I blink hard trying to clear the cloud. My body starts to shake. What do I do? Why can't I see? Am I just tired? What's going on? I slam on the brakes but it's too late.

CRRRRRRRRRRSHHHHHHHH . . .

I crash into the car in front of me. I somehow manage to put the car in park. The fog in my eyes turns into tears.

7

My Turn to Choose

THIS ISN'T RIGHT

I PULL OUT THE "Tuesday Morning" box from my medicine organizer, pour a glass of milk and sit at the kitchen table. Time for my morning cocktail.

Every Sunday night Mom pulls out all of my pill bottles and the empty organizer. She opens the twenty-one little plastic boxes that are marked for each day and whether it's "Morning," "Afternoon," or "Evening," and then fills each one with their special mix of medications. She fills them all; I swallow them all.

I lay this morning's cocktail of eight pills out on the table next to my milk. Some are round; some are capsules. They create a colorful rainbow: red, pink, white, blue. There are five pills in my "Evening" boxes. Add this together with the one yellow pill I take in the afternoon when I visit the nurse and this makes fourteen pills daily. It's my all-time high.

The words "chemical imbalance" ring through my head as I look at the pills. This is how they explain what is wrong with me. I'm not crazy: just imbalanced. It's all a matter of chemistry.

The first sip of milk is my favorite: the creamy texture, the cold temperature. My stomach churns as I pick up my first pill. I grimace, knowing that each one is supposed to add something to my chemistry to balance me out. Why do they have to wreak such havoc on my body?

Down they go, one at a time, each with its own chaser of milk. I see the familiar frown on Mom's face as she watches me from the kitchen counter. She hates watching me swallow these pills almost as much as I hate taking them. I finish my last pill, drain my glass and get up from the table.

As I pass Mom I notice her vanilla folder on the counter. This is my "medication file" where she keeps track of all the different medications I'm on and other details related to my diagnosis.

There's a chart lying on top of the folder I've never seen before. I recognize her handwriting and the names of the drugs. She's also drawn in all these different lines connecting the names together.

"What's this?" I ask.

"It's a diagram of your medicines. I've connected all the drugs to their side effects and then connected the side effects to the drugs prescribed to counteract them. Lithium on this side creates acne so then we zag over here to the acne medication which adds to your tremors so we zig over here to the medicine to stop the tremors which causes your hair to fall out so we zag over here..."

Her voice falls away as her eyes meet mine. For a moment neither one of us knows what to say.

"This isn't right, Lauren." She tucks the chart into the folder and announces, "I've already faxed this chart to Dr. B but haven't heard anything from her. I'm going to show it to her tomorrow. Something needs to change."

DR. B's RECOMMENDATION

MOM MEANS BUSINESS THIS TIME. Her jaw is set and she has her vanilla folder tucked under her arm like she is carrying the world's most important document. We walk quietly up the steep narrow stairs to Dr. B's office. She is the fifth shrink I've seen in the last four years. A family friend whose child is having similar "issues" recommended her. She is supposed to be good at correcting chemical imbalances. So far all she has done is add more pills to my cocktail.

Mom has tried to talk to Dr. B before with no success. I'm eighteen now and legally an adult. This means that the doctor isn't obligated to speak to my parents about anything. She tells my mother this frequently and has frozen her out of my care. She also points out that I have to learn to handle my medications and "manage" myself with college coming up soon. "True enough," Mom says, but I can tell the lack of control and involvement bother her.

We sit in the lobby for only a moment before Dr. B comes to get me. "Lauren, I'm ready for you." She says as she nods to acknowledge my mother.

"I have some concerns . . . " Mom starts to say.

"Mrs. Polly, I've told you before. Lauren needs to bring the concerns to me herself. You can't play the mediator anymore."

"Did you get my fax?" Mom asks as Dr. B leads me away from her.

"Yes, I'll review it with Lauren and then get back to you." She says over her shoulder.

We enter her office and sit facing each other in comfy leather couches. Something is different today: I don't know if it's the chart that I saw yesterday or the way Dr. B is sitting in her chair. I sit up straight and keep my eyes fixed on her.

"Your mother has been faxing me updates on your care. She sent me the graph she made of the medicines. She's rightfully concerned over the side effects and your recent car accident."

Ever since the car accident the worry ripples I feel from my mom are even stronger. It's not just my acne, dry mouth, loss of hair, explosive bowels and tremors anymore. Those were bad enough. The loss of my vision and a car crash? Not okay.

I nod my head like I'm used to doing in this office. I don't need to speak much. Dr. B likes to run the show.

"I think you should see a specialist in Baltimore for a second opinion on your medications." She pauses and looks at me. She doesn't ask me if I want to go or what I think. I thought I was supposed to be learning how to handle this myself!

Without another word she nods her head sharply and goes and gets Mom. They return together and sit stiffly facing each other. My mom holds the vanilla folder against her chest like armor, ready to use its contents in my defense. Dr. B shares her recommendation that I see a specialist.

"Yes," Mom says, relieved to finally have a new solution. "Yes, as soon as possible."

THE SPECIALIST

ANOTHER SET OF LEATHER sofas in yet another shrink's office.

I sigh as I answer question after question. He's giving me all the usual tests. I follow the whispers like I did the first time I was diagnosed and give .the answers I know he is looking for. I look for the clues on how to act, just like the snake taught me. My extensive research and past performances serve me well.

Before the appointment with the specialist our house was filled with a new energy. Mom didn't frown as much and actually smiled a few times at me as she watched me take my morning cocktails, as though to say, *"It won't always be like this, honey."*

There's a name for this energy: false hope. I know she's excited for me to see the specialist. She wants to be involved again. She hopes he'll give more recommendations not only on my medications but on my diagnosis as well. She actually hopes he'll overturn the bipolar diagnosis.

But I know better. There is no way out. It's too late for that. This is my role, my diagnosis. Who would I be without it?

The specialist finishes his questions and takes a look at his notes. He goes and gets my mom to have her join me on the leather couch. She looks at me with a light in her eyes I haven't seen in a long time. I stare blankly at her, numbing myself out so as not to feel her inevitable disappointment.

"It is clear to me that Lauren suffers from bipolar." My mother deflates like a balloon. Shoulders slumped, air let out, the light in her eyes extinguished. "I do think we can change a lot of her medications though. She's on so many and some aren't necessary. Other dosages may be cut back a little as well."

Mom sits up a bit straighter. At least there's a silver lining in this news. She takes notes as the doctor shares suggestions for how to adjust my medications. She is still the one who fills my organizer every Sunday. Now there will just be fewer pills to choke down each day.

"These changes should hopefully take away a lot of the side effects."

"Good." Mom and I say in unison.

"And Lauren, I would like you to have weekly therapy before you leave for college next year. I think it is time you reflect on your obsessive drives and how to make choices that will keep you healthy and balanced."

I stifle a laugh at that. Oh good, more talking, just what I need. And what obsessive drives?

The specialist takes a deep breath and looks kindly but directly at my mother. Something else is coming: why is he so serious?

"I do agree with Dr. B that it is time for Lauren to become more involved in her own care. Up until this point you have been heavily involved in her medical management. I think we need to begin helping Lauren prepare for being independent with her medical decisions, especially with college coming up."

Mom and I look at each other. Her eyes are open wide. She mirrors to me the surprise I feel. The invisible umbilical cord pulses between us. It's time to let go. We both know it. But what will happen when we disconnect?

I GET TO CHOOSE

MOM AND I WALK out of the specialist's office into the cool fall Maryland air. We both wrap our scarfs around our necks and hug our arms to our chests. We watch each other make the same movement at the same time and giggle.

"Want to go for lunch?"

I smile and nod, knowing where we are headed: our favorite seafood restaurant in Baltimore's inner harbor. It's where we always go when we are in this area. Usually we are here for baseball games with Drew and Dad. But today it is just us girls.

We walk to the restaurant in silence. I remember when I was a little girl I used to hold Mom's hand as we walked down the street. I smile now remembering how safe I felt with her hand wrapped around mine. We don't talk until we are seated at a big oak table overlooking the silvery harbor.

"What do you think?" Mom asks me as she takes off her coat and settles in. I don't know how to respond. What is there to think?

"I like that he is changing my medicines. I don't like taking that one that can paralyze my face," I answer, rubbing my hands together for warmth.

"Yeah, I never liked you taking that to begin with," her jaw clenches slightly.

"I think we need to look at other options. This doctor seemed to know so much more than Dr. B. Would you be willing to switch doctors to try to find someone better?"

This is the first time I've been asked for my opinion. Over the past four years my doctors and parents have made just about every decision required. I look away from Mom and out the windows. What do I want to do? A rush of energy moves through me.

Even though Dr. B is annoying and I know another doctor could help me more, the thought of having to start from scratch with a new doctor feels exhausting. I'm tired of re-telling my sad tale and having to re-live everything. I don't have the energy for that.

Plus now I will have to start going to therapy weekly again at the specialist's recommendation. That's already another new person to have to play catch up with.

"I would have to start all over again. And I'm going to have to do that next year anyway when I go to college."

"Yes but what about this year?"

We are interrupted by the waitress who sets down steaming bowls of lobster bisque in front of us. I use the interruption as an excuse to pause the conversation. I blow on the soup and watch the steam rise. I smell the sweet scent of sherry as I reach for a piece of sourdough bread.

What about this year? Do I really want to stay with Dr. B? After meeting with the specialist it is clear that she is mismanaging me. He's taking me off some meds and reducing others just after one visit. I've been with her for over a year on the same dosage. I catch Mom staring at me, watching and waiting for me to bring up the subject again.

"It's my choice?" I ask.

"Yes. The doctors are right, you are old enough now to choose."

We eat in silence as the invisible umbilical cord between us expands and contracts, pulling us closer together and then pushing us apart.

"I want to stay with Dr. B."

The cord snaps so abruptly I fight an urge to lunge towards Mom. I see the disappointment in her eyes and watch her swallow words of protest.

She nods her head and finally says, "Okay, it's your call."

And with that, the cord is cut. I lean forward and back, forward and back in my seat. I feel her wavering too. I lean back into my chair and force myself to look away from her and out into the harbor.

What now?

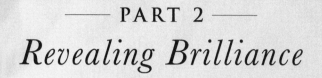

--- **PART 2** ---

Revealing Brilliance

8

Searching for My Place

THE YO-YO SEMESTER

BOOM BOOM BOOM.

The techno rhythm ripples through my body. I dance to the music, tossing my head around so I can feel my hair swing side to side. The air is so stale in here! I throw open the dorm door and drink in the fresh air that comes streaming in. I strip my pants off and spin around with my arms wide out. I love the sensation of the air lifting my oversize t-shirt away from my chest.

"Lauren?"

My roommate in the doorway drags me out of my twirling. Her body is a blur. Her face comes into focus just as I see her raise her eyebrows at me. "The door is wide open, Lauren, and you don't have pants on."

"Yeah, it was suffocating in here with the door closed, Megan. Even my pants felt too tight."

"Okay. Just know that our room is becoming popular with your dance shows." She pushes the door partially closed behind her to so the passing co-eds won't see me. "Just be careful when you are dancing around like that."

I pull her towards me and start dancing again. All disapproval dissolves as she joins me, giggling. We trip over and then smash several plastic cups leftover from last night's, "Lauren's staying!" party.

Megan stops abruptly. "Lauren, don't you have a class soon?"

I look at my digital clock. The bright red numbers 10:45 shout out at me. Oh shit! Ballet class is at 11:00.

"Aghhhh! Thanks, Megan!" I kiss her on the cheek and look around for my pink tights.

"So, you're still staying? Or have you changed your mind already today? We've had more of these parties than I can count over the past month . . . " She kicks one of the smashed cups out of her way as she plops down on her bed.

"At this moment, yes!" I say, flashing a smile at her. I catch a glimmer of something in her eyes. Is she tired? What is that? It looks familiar . . . Ah, yes, it's like the look I saw in my parents' eyes during high school.

I grab my dance bag and move towards the door. "See you later!" I yell without looking back.

I walk quickly through campus, swinging with the techno song that still reverberates through my body. There's a tug at my attention. I look over my shoulder and see a group of girls from my English class. I freeze in their gaze. The music stops.

An invisible hand slaps me in the face as I recall their whispers and looks in class last week. I was the only one to receive an "A" on a writing project. The teacher had me read my writing out loud. The pride I had felt at being acknowledged disappeared with the hot pinpricks of everyone's eyes on me. I shrank in my seat, my face getting hot, and I squeaked out the words that suddenly sounded empty.

My face flushes again as I remember this. I turn away from the girls and continue towards class. With my eyes focused on the path right in front of me I almost bump into Dawn.

"Hey Lauren! Headed to class?"

I look up at her. "Hi . . . yes . . . dance class." Dance class. Safe zone. I smile into her big brown eyes as she loops her arm in mine and we head off to class together.

As we enter the studio I look around at the wall of mirrors and other students in tights, smiling at it all as if greeting a friend. I leave behind the girls' gaze from campus and slip on my ballet shoes. I take my place at the barre and put my hand on its soft polished wood. This, I know. This is my place.

"Lauren? Will you demonstrate a front attitude balance for the class?" the teacher calls out. My belly flips. Again? Another request to be in the spotlight?

All eyes are on me. But this time, my face doesn't flush. Their attention is different. I can sense their admiration and curiosity. What might they learn from me in this pose?

With my left hand still on the barre I shift my weight into my left leg, rising onto pointe while simultaneously lifting my right leg up into a soft curve. I raise my right hand above my head in a matching arch.

"Beautiful, Lauren," the teacher calls. "Now balance."

I let go of the barre with my left hand and raise it to complete the circle above my head. I hold steady as applause fills the room. I ride the wave of appreciation and extend my right leg to its full length and pause, slowly bringing it down in front of my left toe. I come off pointe and close the pose, meeting my teacher's eyes.

"Wonderful. Let's continue." She has everyone take the front attitude pose and then balance. Some students are able to hold it for a moment while others wobble a bit. There isn't any judgment here, though. I smile at my reflection in the mirror as I look around the room. I like this class. I like this teacher. I'm glad I'm staying in college.

We flow through a series of other poses and dance sequences. As the last sounds of music fade, we curtsy one final time. An older student walks over to me as I'm changing my shoes. "Lauren, right?" I recognize her from the posters around campus: she's the lead in the upcoming ballet.

"Yes. Hi."

"You are really good. That was a beautiful attitude hold." She smiles and then moves away. I smile at her back. If I stick around long enough could I be the lead in a future ballet?

I step out of the studio and the jumble of students press against me. I pull my cover-up down as far as it will stretch and move away from their loud conversations.

My belly grumbles and I realize I never ate breakfast. I wonder what they're serving for lunch? Just then I pass the gray brick building of the cafeteria. Whispers fill my ears. They increase in volume until they are screaming at me.

I rake my fingernails over my arms. But I'm really hungry. . . I take a few steps towards the cafeteria and my head explodes in a loud whoosh. I turn and walk away. I can't do it. I can't.

The path blurs in front of me but I don't let my tears stop me. I break into a run and don't stop until I reach my dorm room: my womb room, I once joked with Megan. I unlock the door and this time, close it behind me. The room is empty. No music playing. Crushed cups are still on the floor.

I grab the phone. She picks up after the first ring.

"ERA Realtors. Can I help you?"

"Carolyn? It's Lauren. I need to talk to my mom."

"Ah. Hi Lauren. We were wondering what time you'd call today. It's a bit later than usual."

"Is she there?"

"Yes, hold on." She doesn't bother to conceal the irritation in her voice.

"Hi, honey, you okay?" my mom's voice flows into my ear.

"I can't eat here! I can't go into the cafeteria—it's too loud!"

"I thought you had figured this out. I thought you were going at off times when most people had already gone and left?"

"I am, but I can't on Tuesdays 'cause of ballet class."

"Lauren, you have to eat. Next to sleeping it is the most important thing to staying stable. You know that."

"I do. But I can't go in there!"

"Okay. Where else can you get food?"

"I could drive somewhere . . . "

"Good. Go to a restaurant and get a good meal. When do you see your doctor next?"

"Next week. He said I might have a rough week since he reduced my meds."

"Well, I think you are seeing that now. Please eat and sleep and keep in touch with him and me."

"I think I want to come home. I don't want to stay here."

I hear her sigh before she has a chance to stop it. "Lauren, we talk about this every day. You need to finish the semester. You only have a month left. Can you do that?"

One month. Four weeks. Can I do it? "Yes. I can do that. But I want to come home after."

"Okay. Why don't you go eat something and we'll talk about this later when you are feeling better."

I hang up and sink into my bed, tucking my knees into my chest. The mattress lifts up around me like a hot dog bun. I look over at my car keys hanging by the door. They look miles away from me. How can I ever cross the gap and get my keys, let alone drive somewhere to get food?

I look over at my bedside table. The remote is much closer. I grab it and turn on the television. My hunger and everything else fades away as the happy faces of Monica and Rachel fill the screen. Nothing like a re-run of *Friends* to save the day.

FAILED LAUNCH

"HOW'S IT GOING BEING back at home after leaving college?"

"I didn't leave college," I bark at my new therapist. "I'm still a full-time student, I just transferred to the local university so I could live at home." I squeeze my hands into fists.

Carol smiles at me. "I know, Lauren. I meant how is it living back at home with your parents after living in a dorm for a few months?"

How is it? I ask myself. How do you think it is? I shriek silently. It sucks. It's irritating. It's wrong.

"My parents love me and they are worried about me. I don't fit there anymore. I shouldn't be there at this point in my life and we all know this."

"How so?"

I lean back into the couch, imagining my exhale is a long hiss of steam that hits Carol in the face. A friend from class was telling me the other day how "cool" she thinks it is that I've been going to therapy for so many years. "It must feel great to talk about everything!" she had said. "I have two words for you," I had told her,

"Invasive and irritating!" I look at the clock: how much longer before I can go?

"Lauren?"

"Yes? Oh, sorry. It's agitating to talk about this."

"I can see that. Why?" Bitch. I want to hiss at her again.

"I'm a failure. Everyone else went off to college and did fine. I couldn't handle it. But I don't belong at home either. It's not natural to be at home at this age. But I don't know what else to do . . . "

"How's school?"

"College is fine. The classes are smaller here. I still can't go into the cafeteria. There are too many people there. But I can leave campus whenever I want, so I just leave when I want to eat."

"Is that working?"

"For now."

"Friends?"

"A few. Dance class is fun and I like the people there. I don't hang out with anyone. I usually go home and watch TV."

"How is it with your parents? Did you do the art therapy project I asked you to?"

I reach into my bag and pull out the two sheets of paper with drawings of my relationships with my mom and dad.

"This is my dad's drawing." I lay it out on the coffee table between us. We both look at the mainly blank page with one single image of a black pedestal that has a triangle on top of it. The pedestal is tipping to the side and the triangle has quills sticking out of it.

"Interesting. Tell me about it."

"He is the triangle sitting on top of the pedestal. He is prickly and judging me."

"Has this always been your relationship?"

"No. It's different since I've come back home. We both know that I don't belong there. We are sharp with each other. It's not easy between us like it was before."

"Okay. Let's see your mom's."

I lay out the second sheet on top of Dad's picture. This one is full of color. I lean over to take in the image of a house surrounded by a blooming garden. In the puffy clouds there are huge hazel eyes peering down at everything.

"Tell me about this one."

"It's calm and safe. It's the perfect house on a beautiful spring day. But my mom is watching everything. You can't get away."

"How do you mean?"

I place my hands on the edge of the paper, creating a bit of a frame around it. I look up at Carol. "She checks up on me. Making sure I go to class. Making sure I come here. I have no independence. But then again I couldn't handle being independent at college."

I fall back into the couch with a loud sigh. "We are all stuck not knowing how this is supposed to go."

"Stuck is a good word. Seems like you and your mom might be stuck in an old pattern from when you were younger. She sent me a fax this morning. Did she tell you?"

"What?"

"She sent me a fax about you, telling me about your behavior at home. She says she wasn't sure you would be honest about what was going on, so she wanted to be sure I knew."

I bolt upright. Heat rushes up my spine and floods my cheeks as I look at the many-paged fax Carol hands to me. My mother wasn't sure I would be honest? There are those eyes again, peering right down into my therapist's office. She doesn't trust me . . .

"How does this make you feel?" Another annoying therapy question.

"Pissed."

"It's clear that all of you are struggling. It's awkward for all families who have adult children move back home. You're struggling to find your independence; there are new dynamics and old patterns. Add in your history of mental issues and how difficult it was for you to live away from home and it gets even more complicated."

"So what can we do? I feel suffocated. They are so concerned about me. I know I need to leave but I don't know how to . . . I don't know where to go or what to do."

"Give it time. There will be an opening. Yes, you will have to leave. You can also explore options: where can you go where you'll feel more supported? What would you like your future to be?"

I put the fax onto the table and drop my head into my hands. These questions are exhausting. When will this opening happen? Where is the lifeline I can grab hold of to pull myself out of here?

Mom's voice floats through my head, "We all need roots and wings to succeed."

Forget about the wings! And how the hell can I have roots when I can't even stand on my own two feet?

FLYING TO FANTASY LAND

"LAUREN! IT'S HERE!" FINALLY! I've been waiting weeks to hear from them. Are they throwing me a lifeline or the ax?

I slide across the kitchen floor in my sock feet and stop at the counter where Mom is. She holds out an envelope to me. The Mickey Mouse ears on the envelope tell me it's from the Walt Disney College Program in Orlando.

We smile at each other. In that moment all of our family vacations at Walt Disney collage together in my mind: Dad dancing around in Goofy ears, Drew wearing his favorite Tigger shirt, Mom screaming with joy on the roller coasters. It really is the happiest place on earth.

"This is it . . . " I whisper to her, not quite ready to open the envelope or even take it from her hand.

It was just last month when I saw the small flyer for auditions: "Come work at Disney. Earn college credit. Free housing. Work experience in the park. Meet other students from around the world!"

The moment I saw the flyer, my heart started pounding. Could this be the way out I'd been looking for? Sunny skies, a clear path forward out of the stagnancy of living at home and a brand new start.

The audition was a breeze. All my training in dance and theater, not to mention the doctors' offices, came in handy. I knew how to give them what they wanted so I could get what I wanted. And I wanted this badly.

I had walked into the small classroom being used for the auditions and put on my biggest smile. I shook their hands, looked them straight in the eyes and told them how pleased I was to be there. I regaled them with stories of my happy childhood adventures at the park.

I was the epitome of Disney perkiness! This cheery, chatty behavior was something I had observed during my visits to the park. I also matched the energy of the happy-go-lucky brunette who sat right across from me and asked most of the questions.

"Lauren, I see that you are a dancer and an actress!" she had exclaimed.

"Yes. I've been dancing and performing on stage since I was three and have done a few commercials and print ads. I love being on stage." I paused as I saw her excitement growing. "I've always wanted to dance at Disney," I added, sensing that this comment would open the door I could see was already slightly ajar in her mind. It worked. The door swung open and the information I needed poured out of her mouth.

"That's great! A lot of the college program students come down for the winter semester and then audition and stay to dance for the summer before heading back to school in the fall!" I could tell she was thrilled that she had found a potential longer-term employee in me.

"That's exactly what I would like to do," I responded, smiling in return.

My mom and the envelope come into view again. I take the envelope.

"It's thin," I observe.

We share a look: thin envelopes mean you weren't accepted. We learned this from college applications.

"No matter what, it'll be okay," she says with a little more force than necessary. "Just open it, Lauren."

I exhale loudly as I break the seal. More Mickey Mouse heads greet me as I unfold the paper. "Congratulations, Lauren, and Welcome to the Disney Family!" I read out loud. I barely get the first sentence out before Mom's whooping and clapping drown out my words.

"You got in! Yes! I knew you would!" She grabs me and we jump up and down together. Tears flow down both of our faces. She knew I could. She always believes in me. We stop jumping. As I press my face against her shoulder and feel her arms around me, I recall my first modeling audition when I was fifteen. It was my first audition after my suicide attempt; after the trip to the mental hospital; in the midst of intensive therapy. I had walked out of the theater full of agents with a fake sad face to where Mom was waiting for me. I could see her attempting to hide her hope and worry. And then I couldn't hold it in anymore and I burst out, "I got signed. They loved me!"

She embraced me then like she is hugging me now, jumping with joy that her baby bird has found her wings at last.

Here we go. Time to fly.

HOLISTIC PSYCHIATRY

"MOM! YOU DON'T UNDERSTAND! It's too hard. There is too much to do. I . . . it's . . . it's just so much . . . " I cry into the phone as I twist the long cord around my fingers. I curl up into a corner of the air mattress that is doubling as my bed and couch.

I grab a tissue, wipe my tears and blow my nose. Setting up utilities, paying bills, going on job interviews and managing a house . . . it's all so much. I feel buried with the weight of it. Choosing to stay in Florida after the Disney program ended seemed like a great idea, until now.

I put my hand on my belly. I feel queasy all of a sudden. Did I remember to eat breakfast?

"Mom, what do I do?"

"Lauren," Mom says in her soft voice. If I were standing in front of her right now she would take my hand and look me straight in the eyes. But I'm not there with her, that's why we're having this conversation. I'm supposed to be able to take care of myself.

"You make a list of what you need to do. Then start at the top and work your way down. This is what everyone has to do when they get older. You can do it. Just go slowly and take it one thing at a time."

"Fine," I exhale my irritation and look around my mostly unfurnished apartment. How am I going to furnish this place? What do I need? Where do I go to get it?

A wave of nausea makes me swallow hard. I grip the phone tighter in my hand, wishing she were here with me.

"Lauren," Mom says again. The sound of her voice feels like peppermint tea for my belly. The nausea lessens. "Lauren . . . look at what you've done already. You moved to a new state all by yourself. You've met new people and made new friends. You excelled at your program. If you did all that, you can certainly do these next simple tasks."

I lean against the wall and release my breath as I take in her words. She's right. Who would have thought I could do this all on my own? Me—the one who barely lasted a semester away at college?

The roses on the table catch my attention. They were a gift from Mark. Who imagined I would fall in love, too? He was the one who convinced me to stay after my program ended rather than return home to find a job. I sit up straighter. If I did all of that, what's a few phone calls?

"Maybe your first task could be finding a new doctor," Mom suggests gently.

"All right, Mom. You're right. One thing at a time. I'll find a doctor. Thank you."

We say goodbye and I hang up, resting my hand on the phone for a moment, imagining it's her hand in mine. I pull the heavy phone book up off the floor and drop it on my lap. I flip to the 'P' section to find my new psychiatrist. There are hundreds of listings! Page after page of them. How will I choose?

Another wave of nausea moves up from my belly to my throat. My cheeks feel hot. My hands tremble. The names and numbers blur together on the pages. Who will I choose? All I need to do is pick one. Start with one and see how it goes.

A green box pops off the page. "Holistic Psychiatry," it reads. Holistic. What is that? I don't know what it means but I like the sound of it. It's different.

I pick up the phone and dial the number. "Hello. Yes, I'd like to make an appointment with the doctor as soon as possible. I recently moved here and need to be managed for my bipolar problem."

We make an appointment for the next day. As I hang up the phone, I feel a lightness in my chest. The nausea has faded. Task #1 on my to-do list is done. I take a deep breath. What will this new doctor be like? I get up off my air mattress to make breakfast.

THE SHRINK WHO CHANGED EVERYTHING

MY HANDS SHAKE AS I put my car keys in my purse. Driving on the freeway is still new to me. This is the first time I've driven so far across the city by myself. Only two wrong turns. Not bad.

My belly does a flip. Now that the drive is over I can focus on meeting Dr. T for the first time. I've met so many doctors over the last several years. Will he be any different?

I enter the waiting room and sit down. I look at the empty chairs, recalling all the times Mom used to sit with me as we waited for the doctor. But no more watching eyes. I'm on my own now. I can do this. I grip my purse closer to me and swallow hard to try and dissolve the lump in my throat.

As I look over at the closed door of what I assume is Dr. T's office, it opens.

"Lauren?" he greets me. Wow. He's tall. I nod automatically.

"Stupid question, huh? Who else would you be?" He laughs.

I pause, surprised by his humor and then giggle with him. I usually don't laugh at these appointments. The few times I laughed in the past the doctors looked closely at me, pausing with whatever they were writing in their charts, on the lookout for a manic episode. I could always sense their relief when I squashed the bubbles and didn't let any more surface.

"Come on in," Dr. T says and holds the door open for me to walk past him. I take a few steps into his office and then pause.

"Have a seat wherever you want."

I move to a cushioned leather chair and sit on the edge. I gaze over at his bookshelves filled with what must be hundreds of books. I can make out some of the titles: *Holistic Healing, Energy Medicine, Nutrition for Health.* These books and titles are different from the boring gray books the other doctors had in their offices.

I look around at the rest of his office. It looks more like a living room than an office: a fancy rug, a big oak desk and art on the walls. The painting behind his desk of a Native American riding his horse captures my attention. The young man is staring behind me at some destination, looking determined to get there.

"Do you like the painting?"

"Yes. My dad likes Native American art and my aunt used to live in Arizona. The painting behind your desk reminds me of what I saw in galleries there."

"I bought that one in Arizona when I was there for a conference several years ago." We both gaze at the painting for a few more moments. Then Dr. T sits down in a chair next to me, not behind his desk, and asks, "So, Lauren, what can I help you with?"

"I'm bipolar."

He looks at me in silence, inviting me to continue.

"I'm on medications and need someone to follow me to make sure everything is okay. You know, the basic stuff."

"Okay. I can do that. But I work differently than other doctors. I like taking a more holistic approach."

"Yes, I saw that in your ad. What does that mean?"

"I don't like doing just medication checks. Seeing someone twice a month for 10 to15 minutes isn't the way to really address what is going on for someone. So I do hour-long sessions. I combine medicine management with therapy and holistic modalities for your whole body." He pauses. I take in a deep breath. Holistic. Hmmm. Definitely different.

"What are holistic modalities?"

"I include nutrition, exercise, stress relief practices and personality testing and development. It's more than the medications, Lauren, so much more than that. If you like the sound of this and we continue to work together, we will create a plan that will help develop all of you. That way we can set you up for success in life."

Success. No doctor has ever mentioned that word to me before. They've used words like stable and safe, but never success. I put my hand on my thudding heart. Is success even possible with a bipolar diagnosis? I nod at his words, not able to say anything.

"What do you think?"

"I'm not sure yet." I stare at this new doctor I have chosen, who is so different than others I have seen. "I guess we can try."

---- 9 ----

I Don't Belong Here

DREAM HOME

"YOU DON'T GET IT LAUREN," Mark snaps at me as we wait in line at the town hall. "To these people you don't exist."

My words get caught in my throat and I have to push them out, but they sound quiet even to me, "I do exist. I'm here."

"I was the one who put the money down for the house. That's all they care about. You don't have any money so, no, you don't exist here. Not to them anyway."

I look around at the older people in suits bidding on the empty lots. If we get selected in the lottery, we will be able to build our dream house in the most perfect place on earth: Disney's residential neighborhood.

I tug at my shorts and wiggle my toes in my flip-flops. My belly churns. He's right: I don't exist to anyone here. Although we both work at the park, I work an hourly job and Mark has a management job. I don't have the money it takes to invest in a house. I curl in closer to Mark and slip my hand into his. I catch his eye and give him a small smile, squeezing his hand.

"God, Lauren," he whispers, "Why do you always cling to me like this in public?" He pulls his hand from mine and takes a small step away from me. I look down at my toes, suddenly frozen in place. I tuck my hands in my armpits. "He's just nervous," I tell myself. "He really wants this house. It's a lot of money but he really wants this for us."

I sneak a look back up at Mark. He's staring straight ahead. I want to reach up and touch his brown hair that's cut short, but I press my arms in close to my sides, not daring to let my hands escape my armpits. *"Don't talk. Just look pretty,"* he once told me at a dinner with his colleagues. My face gets hot at this memory and I look away.

My roommate was the one who introduced us. I couldn't believe he was interested in going out with me. He was total husband material: gorgeous, great job, college graduate. On our first date at a fancy dinner he told me he had money saved up for an engagement ring for his wife-to-be.

After two months of dating, during which he surprised me with expensive gifts and weekend getaways at luxurious retreats, he invited me to move in with him. Even though my parents referred to us now as, "shacking up," I loved playing house with Mark. Except in moments like these.

I smile as I remember how he celebrated me on my twenty-first birthday last month. It started with a note telling me to be ready to go by 5 pm when he got off work. He also included a list of what to pack for this surprise trip. All day I was so excited, wondering where he was going to take me.

When he got home he blindfolded me and drove us to our destination: a fancy beach resort on Vero Beach. Our room had a king-size bed and amazing views of the ocean. When I emerged from the shower he surprised me again with a large gift-wrapped box. In it was a fancy dress I had admired months ago in a shop in Epcot. I didn't have words to thank him for his kindness and generosity, just kisses.

I felt like a princess that night as I wore my dress and we feasted on lobster and steak. Afterwards we went dancing and took a long walk on the beach, holding hands and pausing to kiss and stargaze.

Suddenly, I'm sucked back into the town hall. "We got it!" Mark yells. I smile up at him, excited by his excitement. And I wait for a clue: is he going to include me?

He answers my unspoken question by pulling me towards him in a big hug. Then he grabs my hand and leads me up to the front of the room to collect our prize. Everyone is clapping. I smile up at Mark, unable to look at the audience of suits. He smiles down at me and then looks out at the room full of people.

This time, as I squeeze his hand, he squeezes back. He looks down at me again, "We've got our dream home, Lauren. It's ours."

REALITY BITES

HUNCHED OVER MY HANDLEBARS, I pedal quickly down the smooth pavement of our dream home driveway. I turn right onto the sidewalk and race to the nearest cross street. As I take another right turn I look over and see Mark's car pulling into our driveway. I escaped in the nick of time.

I continue to ride fast along the suburban streets. Now that I'm safely out of range of the house I sit up straight and breathe in the scent of orange trees and freshly mown grass. The cool evening breeze strokes my bare arms; it is a welcome treat to the heat of the day.

I tell myself I'm not sneaking away; after four hours of classes and six hours at work, I just want some space to myself.

As I take a left turn to head towards my favorite lake, I realize I've gone on bike rides almost every night so far this month. Except on the nights Mark worked late. On those nights, the moment I heard the garage door open, I turned off the television and jumped into my side of the bed, pretending to be asleep when he came upstairs.

I lift my face up to the sky. The pressure of the thick air on my skin is welcome. I shake my head, recalling Mark's pressure that has become extremely annoying. All he does is push his agenda about marriage, money, future kids, even my doctors. Push, push, push. He doesn't let up.

It's been hard to get clear on what I want when I'm around Mark. All his pressure suffocates me. Thank goodness for Dr. T. He's been helping me pick my way through all of this. His words from our recent session ring through me:

"Lauren, you are at a huge growth place in your life. You are about to graduate college, you have excellent grades and are eyeing graduate schools. You are becoming not just more stable and self-sufficient but successful. Do you really want to limit yourself based on a love that is dwindling?"

A love that is dwindling...

How did that happen? How did Mark go from being my best friend and lover to a stranger? How did we go from planning a future together to now... less than a year later, here I am, wondering about a future for myself, by myself?

As I pedal through our picture-perfect Disney town my mind spins, playing Mark's recent arguments on a loop. His voice slices through the gentle hum of insects, silencing them.

"We can only have one kid—they are too expensive."

"What?" I respond to him freely in my own mind, now that I'm not near him. "How is money the deciding factor in everything we do?"

"You don't help around the house enough."

He's such a jerk. I have a full caseload of classes. I work twenty hours a week at a day-care center. And I've had an ongoing sinus infection for six months. I'm tired. Is it really important to scrub the sink each day so that water spots aren't seen?

"Do you really need a master's degree? Couldn't you just start working after you graduate so we can have more money?"

Do I really need a master's degree? I'm shocked by his question. I'm getting straight A's. My professors have told me I have amazing potential for becoming a speech therapist. I don't want to stop after my bachelor's. I want to go to the best graduate program!

Since my college here is losing accreditation for its master's program, I've been talking about moving a few hours away to go to a better school.

"Lauren, if you move out, that is it. If you leave we are done. We won't survive long distance."

Really? We are planning to spend the rest of our lives together! We can't be a few hours away for two short years?

"I don't have the money to pay for the house by myself. You are selfish for putting me in that position."

Selfish? Really? What about my future?

When I pointed out that my salary would double with a master's degree, Mark had paused in his argument against going on to graduate school. But not for long. He kept finding other things to pressure me about.

"Your doctor is too expensive. If we get married then you'll probably have to start seeing a less expensive one."

WHAT? I want to shout at him. Are you kidding me? Dr. T has shown me a whole other path for my life! Without him . . . without him . . . I shiver in the warm night. I don't even want to consider what my life would be like without Dr. T's support.

Mark promised me and he even promised Dad that he would provide for me and make sure I keep seeing the best doctors if we got married. And Dr. T is the best.

I laugh, but the sound is hollow. It strikes me as funny—and weird—that the entire father to future son-in-law talk, Dad had with Mark focused on my bipolar disorder. Dad told me later he wanted to make sure I would continue to have everything I needed to be stable. What about having everything I need to be happy?

I reach the lake and get off my bike, gently lowering it down into the green grass. I lift my arms up overhead, stretching side to side. I look around the perimeter of the lake. Nobody else is here tonight. I sigh with relief as I walk over and sit on a large rock by the edge of the water.

The sun and water are playing together, creating orange sparkling patches that ripple and bounce with the waves. A family of ducks swims by. Even though they're gliding by in one line, the mama duck keeps looking back, checking in on her little ones.

Just like Mom and Dad who check in on me. They've always wanted the best for me. I close my eyes and take a few deep breaths like Dr. T has taught me.

I recognize the feeling I'm having with Mark: it's the same suffocated feeling I had when I returned from college to live at home. What's different though is that my parents supported me in leaving home; they wanted me to soar.

I'm stunted in this relationship. There is no room to spread my wings. There is no support to fly. No Master's Degree? No Dr. T? No. This isn't what I want for my future.

I open my eyes and gaze out at the lake. I take another deep breath as I allow myself to realize what's true for me: this relationship isn't working for me. It's time for another change.

MY BREAK FOR FREEDOM

"YOU COULD HEAR a pin drop..."

The phrase circles in my mind as I pick at my cinnamon roll. The sun peeks in through the blinds, making bright lines across our small kitchen table. I look over at Mark.

His red plaid pajama pants and t-shirt are wrinkled from sleep. His hair is tousled; so different from his perfectly combed style for work. He's hunched over his cereal bowl, focused on eating. This was always my favorite time to sit with him: no suit and tie, no agenda. Morning after morning we've sat together at this table. This morning, he looks like a stranger to me. I feel miles away from him.

I look back at my own plate. I can't eat a bite of this roll. Ever since I made the plan to leave my belly has quivered with nausea. I gaze out the window through the slats of the blinds. I see slices of the tree in our front yard. Kind of like my relationship... about to get sliced up.

Today is the big day. Knowing Dad is nearby gives me strength to follow through on my plan. He flew down yesterday and is waiting at a hotel now. When Mark leaves for work, he'll come over and help me pack up and... and... leave.

The secret weighs on my chest. I have to focus on drawing in breath. I look back over at Mark. He doesn't know this is our last breakfast together. I wonder what he would say if he knew? But that's why I haven't told him.

My mind churns along with my belly. I told Dr. T yesterday that I was finally ready to leave but didn't know how to.

I was afraid of how Mark might react. I shared my fear with Dr. T. "Mark once told me that when his college girlfriend cheated on him he threw her against a wall in anger. He told me this when we first started dating, it felt like a threat. I can't believe I didn't see this as a red flag then but now . . . "

"Lauren, people get upset and do things in the heat of the moment that they regret later. Did Mark really mean to hurt his old girlfriend?" Dr. T asked.

"No. He regretted it instantly and felt so bad about it."

"Sounds like his anger got the best of him. How do you think he might respond when you tell him you are leaving?"

I paused for a long moment before admitting, "He might get really mad."

Dr. T nodded and was quiet. Then he asked, "What if you didn't confront him with your decision to leave but instead gave him time alone to process any anger he might feel?"

"What do you mean?"

"What if you leave when he is away so he doesn't have to watch you pack and you don't have to argue about your decision? You can leave a note for him and let him know you are taking time to think about what you want. You can tell him you will call him in a week or so to talk. After that you can meet in a public place to talk and resolve things as needed."

"So this way it's not as abrupt?"

"Yes. Give him time and don't put yourself in any danger where his anger may do things that both of you will regret later."

The plan was hatched. I called my parents right after my session with Dr. T and my dad agreed to fly down immediately to help me.

I'm startled by the sound of Mark's chair scraping across the floor. He gets up without a word and heads to the bedroom to take his shower. I can't stand to be inside any longer, pretending. "I'm going for a walk," I call out to his retreating back.

"Okay. See you after work."

I feel a lump in my throat. "No you won't," I silently respond.

I step outside and try to take a deep breath of the morning air. The lump of tears blocks any deep breathing. I watch the sun rise higher in the sky, beaming through the palm trees. I move down the driveway and turn right to take one last walk around the block. My feet feel like they're not quite touching the ground, like they're ready to lift off. My breath comes easier as I get further away from the house. The churning in my belly turns into a fluttering. Is that excitement? Fear? I put my hand on my belly and lift my face to the sun. I'm doing this.

I circle around the block and instead of returning up the driveway, I stand across the street, staring at the blue and white dream house we built together: the perfect house for the perfect couple. This is everything I had dreamed of; everything I thought I wanted; everything I was supposed to want. Only, it stopped being the perfect life a long time ago.

I'm not the "little woman" Mark wants me to be. I'm no longer willing to "be quiet and look pretty." I want more for my life. I want graduate school. I want a career. I want ME.

I see Mark coming out the front door. I press against the closest palm tree. Luckily, he doesn't see me as he moves towards his car. He looks immaculate as always: cleanly shaven, expensive suit. I open my mouth to call out to him but no sound comes out.

I watch as he drives away. And that's when the tears start to fall. I suck in a breath and stifle a sob at the same time. I rest my wet face in my hands. It's done. The wordless goodbye is over.

Dad. It's time to call him. I lift my head and wipe my face. It's time to pack up. This is it. I'm ready to fly.

SCRAPBOOKING MYSELF TOGETHER

DIRTY DANCING HAS BEEN playing for a while on the screen; I look up from my Oprah magazine just in time to watch Baby (Jennifer Grey) leap off the stage into Johnny's (Patrick Swayze's) sexy arms. I love that scene. Such trust. I sigh and lean back into the couch. Could I do that? Let go of control, and trust like that?

I toss Oprah on my new coffee table. I look at my feet beside the magazine and wiggle my toes in greeting. "These are my toes!" I wiggle them again and pause; wiggle, pause, giggle. I never would have been allowed to put my feet up on the table around Mark. That just wasn't "proper" behavior. No more being proper to please him!

I stroke the sage green fabric of my new couch like I would a cat. "This is my couch," I whisper. I had fallen in love with the curvy shape and color of this couch when furniture shopping with Dad and was so excited to have it in my new home.

In the Dream House, all my stuff had been put in the garage. Mark picked out our furniture, our decorations, everything. *"Nobody puts Baby in a corner,"* I laugh as I remember Patrick Swayze's sexy voice. Nobody puts my stuff in a garage anymore. No more hiding.

I slide off the couch and sit on the beige carpeted floor, pulling my scrapbook onto my lap. I rest my hands on the cover as I remember Dr. T's words, "Engage your creative side. Explore . . . who are you now that you're not in relationship? Who do you want to be? What do you dream about for your future? You have less than one year left of college. You'll start applying to graduate schools in a few months. This is your time, Lauren. What will you create?"

His questions stir up my own. Who am I if I'm not Mark's girlfriend? What will my future be now that I gave up the one that was clearly planned and defined? I don't know. I don't know. *I don't know.*

I open my scrapbook to a blank page and run my hand across its smooth surface. Blank. Empty. Like me.

I reach for the numerous magazine clippings I've already cut out, the quote books I've collected over the years, my old journals and sparkle pens. Armed and ready, I think, to create my life.

A clipping from the pile grabs my attention. It's the title to a Dixie Chicks song. *"Wide Open Spaces"* Yes. That. Wide open spaces. That's my life now; alone, foreign, empty, but a welcome change from the suffocating pressure of being with Mark. I glue the clipping to the top of the page and draw a small rolling green hill below it.

I flip through one of my quote books and Gertrude Stein's wisdom pops out at me: "Every day is a renewal, every morning the daily miracle. The joy you feel is life." —Gertrude Stein. I read the last sentence over and over again, "The joy you feel is life. The joy you feel is life. The joy you feel is life." I write her words at the top of the hill with my gold sparkly pen.

I open one of my journals and find my own words calling to me: "I am in awe of the possibilities I have in front of me." I add that to the page, this time with a blue sparkly pen. I repeat my own quote several times, "I am in awe of the possibilities I have in front of me. I am in awe of the possibilities I have in front of me. I am in awe of the possibilities I have in front of me."

The words blur on the page; the tears gently flowing down my cheeks surprise me. I put my sparkly pen down and let the tears keep flowing. I sob softly. Only these tears are different . . . they aren't tears of missing Mark.

I remember Dad's words when I told him I was finally ready to leave Mark, "Lauren, I'll be right there. I'm coming down to help." I remember Mom's voice echoing Dad's, "We're here for you, Tuey." I remember Dr. T's words, "This is your time, Lauren. What will you create?"

I have so much support and so many possibilities ahead of me. Dr. T is right, too.

I get to dream. I get to create. I don't need to know it all right now. I get to explore.

I remember the energy-tuning class I went to last week at Dr. T's office. We partnered up and took turns lying on massage tables and tuning into each other's 'chakras'. I had never heard about these energy centers before and was amazed to discover I could actually sense energy swirling in my partner's different chakras.

I laugh as I remember Dr. T saying to me, "Relax Lauren, there is nothing you have to do. Just hold your hand there. The energy takes care of the rest."

"But I want to make sure I'm doing it right."

"You are. Just look at how relaxed she is."

I looked down at my partner's face. Her eyes were closed, her face looked relaxed, and she was breathing slowly and steadily. If I can learn about chakras, feel energy in someone else's body like that, and help relax them . . . what else might I be able to do?

I return my attention to my scrapbook. The glue and sparkly-pen writing have dried so I flip through the other pages that I've already filled with quotes, doodles and pictures. I glance down the page that has reflections on high school, the teasing, being bipolar; there's a page about my relationship with Mark; there's a page filled with words describing me: bubbly, wild, strong.

I pause on a page filled with poems and reread one by Robert Frost:

> *"Two roads diverged in a wood, and I,*
> *I took the one less traveled by,*
> *And that has made all the difference."*

Mmmm . . . this is the first time I really feel like I have a say in the two roads. It's totally up to me this time.

I look over at another poem on the page, this one by Maya Angelo, "Every Woman". One of the passages calls out to me:

"A WOMAN SHOULD HAVE a feeling of control over her destiny"

After being so out of control for much of my life, having a sense of control over my destiny is what I most want.

I flip through the pages that capture some of the color and depth of my journey so far. I have more blank pages waiting for me. Which path will I choose? What will I create?

10

Living From the Neck Up

BRAINS OVER BODY

I CAN'T BELIEVE I choked so badly! Forgetting my lines? Groping for words as I stared off into space? I've never done that before in an audition. Never.

I kick a small stone out of my path as I head towards my mailbox on the other side of the apartment complex. My face feels hot. I couldn't even look the agents in the eyes during or after my performance. Yet another failure: "No confidence," they'll mark on their forms.

I aced my auditions for modeling and acting all through high school. I thought it would be the same way again here in college theater. I really wanted this. After Mark . . . well, after Mark, just like after my diagnosis, I need something to give me a boost. I needed this.

And my body! What's going on with my body? I look at my legs covered in denim. My feet are carrying me forward but I can't feel my legs. I look at my chest, covered in a green shirt. What's going on in there?

Just like in the audition. Wooden. Robotic. No more fluid movements like in my dancing days. A scene of me dancing across the stage flashes through my mind. When did I stop being at home in my body?

I come to a standstill in the middle of the path outside the mailbox center. When did I stop dancing? I try to remember how many years it's been since I went to a dance class. Four years? Four years ago. Is that when I became an empty shell?

The question rings through my head as I start walking again and pull my mailbox key from my pocket. I stare at my hand as it turns the key sideways in the lock. I can barely feel my hand: I see the movement but the sensation is gone.

I open my mailbox and pull out two letters. They are both from my college, University of Central Florida. I open one and the first line jumps off the page at me:

"Congratulations, Lauren Polly, on your academic achievements. You have made the Dean's List for the first time!"

The Dean's List? I gasp. I did get straight A's for the past two semesters but I wasn't expecting this. I quickly open the second envelope.

"Congratulations, Lauren Polly! The President of U.C.F. would like to welcome you to the President's Honor Roll for your outstanding academic achievements."

I stare at the letters, taking in the words: Congratulations. Dean's List. President's Honor Roll. Dean's List and the President's Honor Roll.

I have never been rewarded for my brain. Drew was—is—the smart one, the one with all the awards and academic achievements. I was rewarded with applause from an audience after a performance or with a compliment of my beauty.

I look down at my body. My physical form had always been the priority: dance, acting, modeling. Until college. These past few years have changed my priorities. When did my brain suck up all the talent from my body? Is this what being an adult is all about? Is this what it takes to be successful?

I think of Dad. Mom. I think of the president of my college; the president of the United States. Where is their priority? Mind. Brain. Strategy. Intelligence. I take a deep breath in and just like that, I sense the last vestiges of energy in my body float up to my head.

Maybe this is the answer I've been looking for. The Dean's List. The President's Honor Roll. Maybe this is the new stage to perform on.

I Knew You Could Do This!

AFTER FIVE YEARS, five colleges, ten majors and five moves I'm finally doing it! I'm graduating! The ups and downs of all of these changes don't even matter to me now as I run my hands over my polyester gown and adjust my cap that sits precariously on top of my head. What matters is that I DID IT!

I giggle as I recall the specialist in Baltimore who expressed concern about my "obsessive" drives. I'd love to show him the payoff of my obsessive drives: straight A's for three years in a row; on the Dean's List and President's Honor Roll the last several semesters; and I got accepted into graduate school at the prestigious University of Virginia! I guess my obsessive drives aren't so bad after all.

"Lauren!" Emily's blue eyes sparkle at me. "Can you believe it, we're done?!" I laugh as she hugs me exuberantly. Over the

last two years we've spent hours together studying and support-
ing each other through the ups and downs of college.

"I know! I thought this would never come!"

"Are you all packed up?"

"Yep. I'm leaving tomorrow to go home for a few weeks
before starting at U.Va."

A voice over the loudspeaker interrupts us, "Graduates,
please take your places!"

"Find me after the ceremony! I want to meet your family!"
Emily calls over her shoulder as she makes her way to her place
in line. I make my way to the "P" section and file in to the sta-
dium along with the other hundreds of graduating students.

The press of bodies and noise make my head buzz slightly.
A few deep breaths help the buzz go away. I search the bleachers
for my family but can't find them in the droves of people. I sigh
in frustration, blowing my bangs up with my exhale. I give up. I'll
find them after the ceremony.

The president of the college steps up to the microphone to
speak. As his deep voice drones on I drift away, remembering
last night and how my family joined me for the energy-tuning
class at Dr. T's. Even though it was so different from anything
they would ever do on their own, they wanted to see what it was
like after hearing me talk about it so much. And of course, they
wanted to meet the infamous Dr. T.

Another speaker steps up to the microphone. One of the
trustees? I tune her out and return to my memories of last night.
Having my family and Dr. T all in one room . . . I breathe in
deeply, remembering all the care I felt for them and from them.
They have all seen me through so much.

I got to show them all how to find chakras on each other and
tune into energy. Who would have ever thought we'd be doing

that together? Who would have thought I'd be sharing with them something that was so weird to me just a few months ago?

As we left Dr. T's building last night, arms linked together, laughing and gazing up at the sparkling stars, it was like old times . . . only, better than before. Better than ever.

Suddenly there is a row of graduates in black gowns standing in front of me and I realized it's time for the "P" rows to go up on stage and receive our diplomas. As I walk down the aisle I search the faces in each row. Where are they?

I step up onto the stage and focus on the president of the university who is standing mid-stage holding my prize. I pause and lift my shoulders back, standing up a bit straighter. My chest lifts with a sense of pride. The view of the president blurs through my tears. I'm really doing it!

As I walk across the stage I sense a tug to my left. I look over and that's when I see them: Mom, Dad, Drew. They are all standing up, clapping and beaming at me.

Drew opens his mouth in a fake scream and I stifle a giggle. Dad pumps his fists in the air as his blue eyes meet mine. My gaze finally rests on Mom, who is nodding her head slowly as tears fall down her cheeks. I can hear her as clearly as if she were standing next to me whispering in my ear, "*I knew you could do this. I knew it.*" I smile at her and feel my own tears wet on my cheeks.

As I take the diploma from the president and shake his hand, my chest bursts open and I swear I can feel my wings begin to flap.

TIME TO GROW UP

"LAUREN?" I TURN AND see Pastor John smiling at me.

"Hi Pastor John."

"Good to see you. Are you in town for a visit?"

"I'm just here for a week before going to graduate school."

I keep smiling at him, wondering how he'll respond. Lost and fragile Lauren going to graduate school? Who would have imagined?! I stand up a little straighter and continue with the most impressive news, "I got into U.Va."

His eyes widen. It's the same surprised response I've gotten from everyone else I shared this news with. "Wow. That's terrific. You don't just walk into that school," he pauses and looks at me as though witnessing a miracle. "Be sure to tell Rosemary the great news!" And with that he turns towards the stage to begin the service.

Dad's blue eyes flash at me as I take a seat next to him in the red-cushioned pew. "That sure surprised him, huh?" He says, stifling a laugh. "You've been enjoying that haven't you?"

I nod and smile mischievously at him. Yes. I have been enjoying that. I've discovered I actually like doing the unexpected: getting straight A's; being on the Dean's List; getting accepted at one of the top universities in the country.

I would love to share this unexpected news with the doctors who once told me too much stress would be dangerous for me. I bet they would be surprised, too.

They warned me against challenging myself too much. "The shoe could drop at any moment!" They never imagined I could be this successful, normal and stable.

They thought I couldn't handle the pressure. Ha! I sure proved them wrong. What did they know?

Rosemary calls me out of my reverie with her singsong voice, "Lauren! It's so good to see you!" I melt into her as she bends down and wraps me in her arms. Her bright blue eyes meet mine as she releases me from the hug. The familiar warmth that comforted me when I was fourteen spreads from her eyes to my chest.

"Did you hear?" Dad asks her. "Lauren's going to the University of Virginia!" Rosemary's eyes widen as she looks at Dad and then back at me—her expression is one of delight rather than surprise.

"That's wonderful, Lauren. I always knew you would be successful at whatever you chose."

"Thanks. I just had to stop dancing long enough to discover I had a brain!"

"You're not dancing anymore?" This time her eyebrows go in the opposite direction of her delight and her brow wrinkles.

"No. School has been busy and I wanted to focus there. It was time to grow up," I say, sitting up straighter. The music begins and Pastor John asks us to rise from our seats to sing.

"Well, maybe you'll start up again later," Rosemary whispers. "See you after the service." I watch her as she walks away and takes her seat up front.

I look past where Rosemary sits and out the window at the far end of the church.

The trees seem to call to me. Scenes from when I was a teenager and taught bible study for the children run through my mind. "God made the earth, so let's go enjoy it!" I would call out to the kids as I led them out to the playground. I felt more connected out beneath those trees. Moving and playing beyond the confines of these walls, we escaped the pastor's service and created our own conversation with God.

I turn my attention to the screen up front that displays the words for the hymns. It's time to grow up now. I squint, releasing images of the trees and focusing my mind on the words so I can sing along with everyone else.

MY MIND VS. THE YOGA INSTRUCTOR

SHUT UP! I SILENTLY yell at my mind. But it doesn't listen. Instead, it gets louder, competing with the voice of the yoga instructor.

"Inhale your arms overhead and exhale fold to touch your toes," the instructor calls out from the front of the students' gym.

"Prepare materials for clients tomorrow. Test on neuroscience on Friday. Five—yes—FIVE—chapters to read for Speech Pathology Sciences by Monday..." my mind spins.

I exhale loudly. What does it take for my mind to *shut up?* I copy the movements of the people around me. Where is the peace of mind yoga is known for?

"Inhale look up, exhale step back to pushup position."

"Twenty-one hours of advanced classes. Ten hours of clinic, treating clients. Ten hours of Graduate Research Assistant duties."

"Inhale come down to the mat, exhale to downward dog."

I look up, expecting to see a black cloud above my head. Nope. It just feels that way. I gaze back down at the mat as my arms tremble. How long do I have to hold this stupid pose?

I told my psychiatrist about the spinning mind. "Is this related to my bipolar?" I asked him. "Will more symptoms reveal themselves now that I'm under so much stress? When I was a teenager the doctors warned me that too much stress could put me in danger."

But he isn't concerned. He says it's very common for graduate students—especially when carrying a huge workload like I am—to have a racing mind. I thought about my classmates and realized yes, everyone is stressed out. This is the curse of the graduate student. I'm not alone in this. I'm not going crazy. This is normal.

This craziness is normal? This kind of normal sucks. My psychiatrist laughed when I told him this. As I left his office I remembered Dr. T, and how he introduced me to activities that helped me relax my busy mind. That's when I realized it was time for another yoga class.

"Relax into child's pose," the yoga instructor says in her soothing voice.

I look at the woman on the mat next to mine and copy the pose she's in. The body positions are easy enough to duplicate. I just wish I could duplicate the ease of breath and peace of mind that this woman exudes.

Class ends and as I wipe the sweat from my forehead with my towel, I smile at the calm woman next to me. "Isn't it great?" She asks me with a big smile. "I feel so much calmer and centered now. My body feels so open." I copy her serene smile and her calm eyes. Fake it till you make it, right? Maybe if I copy her serenity on the outside, my insides will eventually catch up. I watch her walk out of class. She appears to glide across the floor with her slow movements. It's like nothing could faze her.

I pick up my mat and then copy her movements for a couple of steps. I exhale slowly, imagining the yoga teacher is still guiding me, "Exhale, feel your feet on the ground . . . "

Then my mind chirps loudly, *"Test tomorrow in medical clinic!"* Oh no! I totally forgot! I run out of the gym. No gliding for me. No more feeling my feet on the ground. My spinning mind is in charge once again.

MY BODY: A PRESSURE COOKER AGAIN

I LOOK DOWN AT my khaki pants and white shirt. Shit! I *hate* this outfit! I throw open my closet door. I have nothing to wear.

The red numbers on my bedside clock catch my attention: 6:48. Shit, shit, shit. I'm going to be late.

My shirt is sticking to my armpits. Oh gross. I'm already sweating. This is not the way I want to start the first day of my internship. I wail and cover my face with my hands. Tears and sweat stream down my face.

A hand that seems to belong to someone else rips my shirt off. Buttons fly as another wail pushes its way out of my body. My throat burns as the screams continue. I rake my nails down my arms. Then I see the raised red trails I've made. I curl my hands into fists and yell, "GOD DAMN IT!"

I wiggle out of the pants and kick them across the room. I am shaking uncontrollably. I slump onto the floor of my closet and curl up into a fetal position. I see an image of the hospital in my mind. I have graduated from the student clinic and am going to work at a hospital today. I'm grown up. This behavior is unacceptable.

I hear my own voice whisper to me, "No. No more. Get up Lauren. Get up *now!*"

I breathe deeply, remembering my yoga practice. Breathe in through my nose; breathe out through my mouth. I pull myself up into a sitting position. More deep breathing as my body continues to shake.

I stand up slowly, steadying myself against the wall. I command my body to stop shaking. I can handle this, I tell myself. Just pick something. I reach for my favorite long black skirt and, balancing against the wall, lift one leg at a time to pull it on. I pull out my pink sweater and pull it over my head. My arms quiver a bit as I stretch them into the tight fabric. I slip my feet into my black flats and look at the clock. 6:52. Five minutes wasted on a meltdown. I thought I was through with these!

I head into the kitchen and grab a muffin, my keys, purse and school bags and head for the door. I catch a glimpse of my reflection in the mirror on the way out the door. My mascara has left black trail marks down my cheeks. My eyes are bloodshot and puffy from crying. I gasp. I haven't seen myself like this in so long.

I do more of my yoga breathing: in through the nose, out through the mouth. Fill my belly in between. I push the feeling of disgust down and out of my body and mind. It'll be okay, I tell myself. I can wipe the black off my cheeks at the stoplights and time will take away the puffiness and redness. No one will know but me.

I CAN DO THIS!

MY BELLY CLENCHES AS I approach the therapy room. I can see my patient is already in there. He looks up from his wheel-chair and meets my eyes. The left side of his mouth raises into a smile, the right side doesn't join in: a consequence of his recent stroke.

This is my first patient at the hospital. I pause at the door, trembling, and tell myself, *"You can do this,"* remembering all the patients I've seen over the past year through my work at the stu-dent-run therapy clinic. I take a deep breath and mentally push the panic out. Although my shoulders relax and the jitters in my belly soften, I suddenly feel lonely. I'm confused; my supervisor will be sitting next to me the entire time. I won't be alone.

What is this loneliness? I look at my patient. He's slumped over to his right side. His back curls forward a bit. I've had other stroke patients tell me how lonely they are. Is he feeling lonely? I wonder. I enter the room, taking my seat across from Mr. G and next to my supervisor. I smile at her and turn my attention to my patient.

"Hi. I'm Lauren. I'll be your speech therapist."

"Mmmmmm. Gggrrrrr. Ooooohhh."

I glance over at my supervisor and wonder what she would do now. I recall her confidence and easy nature with patients. She talks to them in a natural conversational tone despite their inability to speak. I remember how the patients seem to be more relaxed with her than they are with other staff members who expect them to speak normally.

I meet his gaze again, focusing on his eyes, not his drooping face. "It's nice to meet you."

"Hhhhhh. Rrrrgggg," he says, leaning forward.

"Okay. We're going to start with you naming some pictures. I know you know what the pictures are. You are just having a hard time saying the word. If you have trouble speaking then I'll help you along. How does that sound?"

"Ooooo. Bbbbbbbb." He nods.

"All right. Let's get started."

I show him picture after picture and he practices his sounds and words. I encourage him with nods and smiles and suggestions for sounding out the words. I cue his recall of the word by prompting him with the first sound. I coach him on how to form the right shapes with his lips and tongue to make the correct sound.

"Oh. Look at the time. We're at the end of the session already. That went fast!"

"Kkkkkkkk," he responds with a nod and a half smile.

"We're going to do this again next week. I'd like you to practice at home with your wife. Okay?"

"Oh. Kay."

I laugh and grin at him. His eyes widen as he tries his best to grin widely back at me. That makes us both shake with laughter. A few bubbles float from my belly out my mouth in more laughter.

"Wow! You just said 'Okay'!"

My bubbles expand and spread to him. As he laughs, the left side of his face rises into the biggest smile yet. Even his right side moves a little. He reaches out his left hand, grabbing my hand. He holds on tight with his fingers as his thumb strokes the back of my hand. I feel a lump in my throat and blink back tears.

"Ttthhhhh. Uh."

"You are welcome." As I watch his wife wheel him out of the clinic, I wipe tears from my cheeks.

"Well done, Lauren," my supervisor says as she stands beside me.

"Wow. I can do this!" The words escape before I have a chance to edit myself.

She laughs. "Yes. Your natural ease with people will serve you well in this field. Take a few minutes to break and then we'll meet up to discuss the session."

I nod and watch her walk away. 'Your natural ease with people . . . ' Who would have thought?

PAVING THE WAY FOR KIDS
(BEFORE I HAVE A HUSBAND)

I CAN SEE THE hospital where I work out the window behind my new shrink's chair. The southern charm of Atlanta delights me—even in the winter the magnolia trees are green! After the cold winters in Virginia, I was delighted to move here to accept a position at a prestigious hospital.

Dr. S takes a seat on the other side of the desk from me, blocking some of the view. I sit up straighter, cross my legs and wrap my fingers together in my lap.

This new doctor looks different than any of the others I've been to: long flowing shirt with flowers on it, blue scarf draped around her neck. She has piles of snacks, a mess of papers and photos of kids on her desk. She seems less formal, more like Dr. T was, though he would have a fit if his office looked this messy!

I gaze at one of the photos of two smiling kids looking up from an art project. They're probably her kids. I smile at the happy faces. I found the right doctor. She is a mom. I want her help managing my psychiatric medications when I become pregnant so I can be a mom, too.

Not that I'm trying to get pregnant now. I'm just one foot ahead of the game like my dad always says. I've met my other goals already. Master's degree. Check. Full-time job at one of the country's best hospitals. Check. My own car. Check. My own house. Check. Next comes the husband and then the kids.

I return my attention to Dr. S as her chair squeaks. She leans back into her chair, looking like she is about to watch a movie, not sit with a patient for the first time. I exhale slowly and loosen my hands from their tight grip on each other. Dr. S picks up a pad of paper and pen, folding a page full of scribbles over to a clean sheet. I suck in my breath. Here we go . . .

"So, Lauren. Can you tell me a little about your history?"

"I'm bipolar. I was diagnosed when I was fourteen. I've done the whole gamut of traditional medications over the years. I was on Lithium, then Depakote and various anti-depressants and anti-anxiety meds mixed in as well. I was also on anti-psychotic meds for a short while in the beginning. Right now I'm only on 300mg of Neurontin and am doing fine."

Dr. S raises an eyebrow as she moves from side to side in her swivel chair. I don't allow myself to get distracted by the movement. My eyes meet her brown ones and hold steady.

"It's unusual to be stable on only that medication and that small a dosage."

"Yes. I've been weaned down by various doctors over the years. I did psychotherapy for about ten years straight and use everything I learned there daily."

"That's good," she says casually, not showing any signs of being pleased that I do what I'm told. She is different than the others. She continues to stare at me calmly. I sit straighter in my chair and press my hands against my blue scrub pants.

"You work here at Emory?"

"Yes. I'm a speech pathologist."

"Why are you wearing scrubs?"

"I work in the ICU with patients with swallowing disorders and tracheostomies." I smile at the slight surprise in her eyes.

"There's a lot of body fluid," I offer to explain my clothing choice.

"Ah. Easier to clean." she smiles in return.

"Yes." I agree with a giggle.

"Emory is an intense environment. And your job in particular sounds quite stressful. How do you manage it?"

"I do fine. I eat well. I make sure to go to bed by 9:30 every night. I don't talk on the telephone after 8 since it's harder to wind down to fall asleep on time if I do. I don't watch TV after that time either."

No praise for my good behavior and managing techniques; only a calm stare and a long pause.

"The expectations at work were hard at first. The pace is faster. And the patients are more complex than anywhere I've worked before. It takes a higher skill set but I'm smart and a fast learner."

"I can see that about you."

"Yes. It serves me well."

"So what is it you require from me?"

"I just need to be followed for my medication at this point. But I also saw that you specialize in helping women manage their psychiatric medications and disorders when they are pregnant."

"Are you thinking about having a baby soon?"

"Well, not so soon. I'm still single but I thought I would like to plan ahead and work with you now so when I do meet my husband we are all set to go."

Her eyebrows lift again as she laughs. "You are on top of things, aren't you?"

I smile, happy to be acknowledged at last. "Yes. I find I do better that way."

"Okay. Here's your prescription for now. I'd like to see you back in three months for a check-in. We'll see how your husband hunting is going then." She winks as she hands me the paper with the familiar words on it: Neurontin 100mg TID.

I smile and turn to leave, staring at the paper. Familiar words, same medicine, same dosage. But there is something different about her and about our work together. Something else just might be possible here.

11

Coming Home to My Body

THE MIND HAS A HEART

"HE DOESN'T WANT YOU. He didn't choose you. You don't matter to him. You don't matter PERIOD." My heartbreak triggered a head-trip. *"You don't matter to him. He didn't choose you. He doesn't want you. You don't matter."*

I think of our first date out on the patio of the restaurant Carpe Diem, our first kiss, the last time we made love . . . I did everything like I was supposed to, everything my friends did to meet and marry their husbands. I chose a man with the same educational background, the same upbringing, the same family values. Why didn't it work out?

Talking to my friends about David's rejection helps a little. But it's not enough. I still can't breathe well. My chest is tight. The words and memories are suffocating me. Jill suggested I go to yoga. "It made you feel a little better in grad school. Remember? Why don't you try it again?"

I pulled out my old leotards that hadn't been worn in three years and, surprised and grateful that they still fit, drove to the closest studio. The overpowering scent of incense greets me at the door. I breathe it in.

I wonder what thoughts or memories I need that would overpower all my memories with David. What would erase the image of his hazel eyes and naked body? What would erase his last words to me, "I'm sorry, Lauren, but I'm just not interested in a relationship." Then maybe, just maybe, I could be free of him.

The slim blond woman at the desk looks up at me as I enter. "Hi! Are you new?"

"Yes. I haven't done yoga in a few years and only did it a few times back then."

"That's fine. This upcoming class is open to all levels. You can move at your own pace and skill level."

I put my shoes and purse in a cubby in the hallway and enter the studio. I'm surprised to see so many people in the room. I remember that serene woman next to me at my last yoga class in graduate school. I totally failed at copying her. I never returned to a yoga class after that.

I pick up a mat and blanket from the stacks in the back of the room and head to the middle row to set up my spot. This way I can copy the people in front of me if I don't know how to do any of the poses. I bend over to touch my toes and barely reach them. My hamstrings tug in resistance.

Music begins to play. What's going on? Love songs? Thoughts of David flood my mind as I blink back tears. My chest constricts.

"Hi everyone. Welcome. I'm Yvonne and I'll be teaching the class tonight. We are going to continue on with February's theme of love and move to some famous love songs."

I squint at this heartless woman. Who would be so insensitive? Doesn't she know that not everyone wants to hear about love? My hands curl into fists as tears roll down my cheeks.

"Breathe, Lauren," I tell myself. "Breathe. It's okay. Just focus on the movements."

I swallow and push the tears down, focusing on her instructions. I watch the people around me and copy their movements. Move, don't think. Move, don't think. Every time thoughts of David enter my mind I return my focus to my body and the pose. Just like Dr. T taught me: redirect the mind. Don't think. Just move.

"Inhale arms overhead. Exhale fold to touch your toes. Inhale look up. Exhale fold."

We move and breathe. Breathe and move. I follow the instructions and match my movements to those around me. My mind quiets.

We move into downward facing dog for what seems like the hundredth time. My arms shake. I breathe in more deeply, trying to use my breath as the instructor has suggested to calm the body. Yet my breath gets stopped in my chest. What is that? It feels like a vise grip around my heart. Like a hand redirecting my blood and breath upwards, unwilling to have it move downwards.

I continue to breathe as deeply as I can, but it's not calming my body. My arms continue to shake as I hold the pose. The grip on my heart begins to loosen. I seize this opening and take a huge breath in, pushing the invisible hand out of my body. My heart gushes a wave of warmth up through my chest and throat. I collapse on the mat, giggling to myself. Bubbles press up from my pelvis. What was that?

Yvonne, the torturous teacher and impeller of love, looks at me in surprise. I wiggle my fingers at her as I giggle and enjoy feeling my breath fill my open chest. After a few more waves of bubbles I join the rest of class in the poses. The love songs no longer bother me. My mind is quiet. Maybe there is more to this yoga after all.

NAKED YOGA

MY ARMS ARE SHAKING. My neck is tight. How long is Gina, our teacher, going to have us hold this damn downward dog pose?

I breathe in through my nose and out my mouth. Damn legs, I think to myself. If my leg muscles were activated the right way I wouldn't be putting so much pressure on my arms. They wouldn't be shaking and I wouldn't have knots in my neck. And my pelvis! My pelvis isn't even tucking under the way it's supposed to in this pose.

Oh the joys of training to be a yoga instructor. Now I know what my body is supposed to be doing to be in alignment, to be doing the poses correctly so the energy can flow. Trouble is, knowing it and doing it are two different things.

"Inhale and with your next exhale lower into plank pose." Thank God. I lower into plank pose and from there Gina guides us through the rest of the vinyasa flow more quickly.

After class I roll up my mat and head out the door. Usually I stop and chat with Gina. I've been in a yoga teacher training with her for almost a year. She's become a mentor. But today I need to get out of here.

I jump into my car, throw my mat in the passenger seat, and take off. I hit the steering wheel with my fist as I drive out of the parking lot. Goddamn it! What happened to the lower part of my body? I can't feel my legs anymore. I can't even feel my pelvis. What the hell happened?

I concentrate on trying to feel the gas pedal under my foot as I drive through the streets. I speed up. My leotard sticks to me in the sweltering heat. This needs to change. Now. How can I tell if I'm doing the poses correctly when I can't feel if my muscles are engaged? "How am I supposed to teach others something I'm struggling with myself?" I yell.

I park in front of my townhouse, pushing the door open and slamming it shut behind me. I look up at my beautiful home and suddenly I feel proud. I look back at my car: a brand new Honda Civic, my dream car. Not a hand-me-down like all my previous cars.

I look at my house again. My house. Paid for by working at one of the top hospitals in the country. And now I'm training to become a yoga instructor. "I can do this," I whisper to myself. I can succeed at anything I put my mind to. I know this now.

I enter the house, kick my shoes off and run up the stairs to my second bedroom, which is reserved for my yoga and meditation practices. "Hi Elsa," I call out to my cat who I know is somewhere in the house, while I roll out my yoga mat.

I step to the front of the mat and wipe the sweat off my face. I glance down at my altar, which holds some of my special objects: my Shiva and Green Tara statues and some leaves and stones I collected from a recent hike. I remember the first principle of Anusara Yoga: Open to Grace. *"'Open to Grace' allows you to open to something bigger. You stop with your pushy small efforts and get to relax into your body, into the universe."*

I take a deep breath in and exhale, shaking my upper body, trying to soften the tight knots between my shoulders. I inhale my arms over head and then exhale as I step back into downward dog. I tuck my chin into my chest so I can see my thighs. Are the muscles activated? I can't tell. I try to feel them but I can't. I spread my toes wide to try to engage the muscles more but I still can't feel them. Goddamn it!

I stand up and peel the sweaty spandex pants off my legs and toss them next to the mat. My spandex top is the next to go. The top sticks to my armpits and face. I yank it off and it flies across the room. I turn to see it land next to Elsa who is watching the show from the doorway.

"I can't tell if my muscles are activating! I need to look to see!" As though I need to explain my behavior and nakedness to her. She blinks and yawns at me.

I exhale deeply and curl my body back into downward dog. I again tuck my chin and look back at my legs as my toes spread. Yes. My quadriceps are active. I can see they are flexed. What about my hamstrings? I can't see them to tell. I push my weight into my left arm and lift my right hand up to feel the back of my thigh. Nope. I press my feet backwards against the mat. Ahh! That's it! I touch my hamstring again and can feel the muscle flexing.

I return my hand to the mat and stay in the pose, focusing on the sensations I now feel in my legs. My muscles are active. I have visual and touch confirmation. Now can I feel it from the inside?

Nothing. My chest tightens and I groan. I continue to try different poses, pausing in each one to check my muscles. I look at every muscle I can and touch the ones I can't see. I look and touch. Touch and look. But I don't feel anything from the inside. I blink back tears.

"Open to grace," I remind myself. I try to soften. I try to relax into my body. But how can I relax into a body I can't feel? I collapse on my mat. Through my tears I see Elsa sitting a few feet away, watching me. I curl into the fetal position resting my head on my arm, meeting her gaze.

She gets up to move close to me. I watch her walk towards me. She moves effortlessly, sensually, slowly. She moves like I used to. I can see each muscle in her body activate even though she is covered in long golden fur. Her green eyes meet mine as she lets out a soft meow. She curls her agile and effortless form next to my naked, sweaty, pushy one. My hand curls into her fur and I exhale, softening at last.

After a few minutes I give Elsa a kiss and stand up on my mat, taking the warrior pose. With my right leg at the front of my mat and my left leg stretched behind me, I reach my arms up to the sky. "Open to grace," I whisper, "No more pushing. Relax."

I close my eyes and soften into the pose. I exhale loudly and as I do I release my weight into the strength of my legs. I stop the struggle and settle into the pose. I'm supported. I can support myself, without effort or strain.

I keep my eyes closed and feel into the pose, from the inside. Active yet relaxed. Strong yet soft. I don't need to look anymore. I open my eyes and look at my cat. "Elsa," I whisper softly, "Look. I'm opening to grace!"

SILENCE INSIDE AND OUT

I TAKE MY SEAT. My limber yoga body folds easily into a cross-legged position as I pull my feet under my thighs. I balance on the edge of a blanket for added comfort and ease in my hips.

My teacher, Paul, rings a bell from where he is seated at the front of the room, signaling the beginning of our afternoon meditation session. We're on Day 2 of a week-long Neelakantha meditation retreat. I close my eyes and sink into the quiet stillness that has become a familiar sanctuary.

Gina's face passes through my mind. She introduced me to this meditation practice shortly after I became a yoga teacher. It sounded a bit intense and weird at first, but I trusted her. I dove into the practice and discovered a new tool for cultivating inner stillness that took me even deeper than my yoga practice.

I acknowledge Gina with a silent thank you and return my attention to my breath. My breath is even and tempered now after daily practice for the last two years. I follow it with soft focused attention and ease any rough patches along the way. I have become a master at controlling my breath and my body.

Through the darkness, the seed of my mantra builds from deep in my mind. I invite it to come forth and present itself. I don't articulate it the way you would a word. It is a whisper, a meaningless sound chosen to be a vibrational match for each meditator.

"Don't force it. Just let it come on its own," I can hear Paul say. It's the beauty of this style. No effort. No force. Just soften. It feels so good and contradictory to how I lived my life up until I discovered this practice. There is no battle here. No fight against my mind, my body. Just the ease of the mantra that quiets my thoughts.

The seed opens in my mind and forms a loose syllable. It repeats itself over and over again. I don't match it to my breath. I don't force it. I don't pronounce it hard. I allow it to be soft and loose.

I smile. Yes. I have mastered this. The mantra gets quieter and fades into a quiet. I drop into darkness. The quiet stillness wraps around me like black velvet.

Paul rings the bell again, signaling the meditation session is over. I unfold my legs and lie on my back in savasana, corpse pose. After a few minutes I wiggle my fingers and toes. I roll over onto my side, savoring the quiet stillness in the room. I open my eyes and see my roommate, Dee, in the same position on the other side of the room. We smile at each other.

No talking is allowed on this retreat. In silence I stand up and make my way to the balcony. I want to see the beautiful view of the California desert. The sun is setting over the mountains in the distance, sending beams of sparkling light over the sandy dunes. The desert is silent, just like my inner world. Finally. There is only stillness inside.

A Name for the Dark Energies

"Like attracts like. So when you play with the darker energies you invite that in." Paul's words rumble through me. Usually, his deep voice is soothing, but today his teaching evokes memories of my earlier years of agony.

Reading the passage in the Bible about the brothers' revenge. Feeling the murderous dark energies enter my body, creeping up my arms and down into the dark seed in my belly. Reading the stories about children being locked in an attic. Being abused. Tormented.

"When you play with these energies you open a door for the creatures known as rakshasas to come in and take over. In the Hindu tradition, these dark energies run your body. You become intertwined with them and don't have the clarity of you anymore."

Scenes of the smoky snake swirling around me, one moment friend, one moment foe, fill my mind. Did I open a door for it to enter me? I shiver. I encouraged it. I engaged with it. Was the smoky snake a rakshasa? Is it still inside of me?

"Meditation can clear these energies. The fire practice you are learning—that we have been focusing on during this retreat—burns away unconsciousness. It purifies you so the darkness can't stay hidden within you." The flickering candles at the base of the golden Shiva statue catch my attention. The light burns, purifies the darkness . . .

So even if I am the one who attracted the smoky snake to me, and other dark energies, I am the one who can purify this energy. I sit up straighter on my cushion and return my gaze to focus on Paul. No more playing with dark energy. No more inviting that in. I am purifying myself and all the seeds of unconsciousness that may still be inside.

"The seventh century tradition that you are studying is rigor-
ous for a reason. Every time you meditate, you dip into the fire
a bit further and burn more unconsciousness out of you. This is
the path to greater consciousness."

"Bring it on," I want to say out loud. But we are still in the
silent portion of our retreat where only the teachers speak. So
I whisper it to myself and slowly close my eyes as the sound of
the gong echoes through the room, signaling the beginning of
another round of meditation.

THE SNAKE REAPPEARS

MY RESOLVE TO PURIFY any seeds of unconsciousness has
strengthened over these past two days. I'm diligent with my practice. I take my seat for the final round of meditation and gaze out
the window. The sun is setting and the sky is filled with clouds
painted shades of pink and red. I glance over at my roommate,
Zadie, to see if she's enjoying this beauty too, but her eyes are
already closed.

I gaze out at the sunset again. I have looked out on this
landscape every day for the past week and in all of my previous
retreats. Although the sky changes color and the light grows and
fades, the view never changes. "But I do," I think to myself with
a smile.

I close my eyes and begin to silently repeat my mantra. The
rhythmic repetition of this single syllable carries me down; down
past the busy-mind, past the calm of my breath, and into a velvet
blackness that wraps around me. My mantra continues to pulse
as if on its own. I melt away.

Prickles on my skin grab my attention. My skin flushes with
heat. What is going on? The soothing black velvet dissolves into
red flames that consume me. My belly pulses so hard it aches.

I can't catch my breath. With my eyes still closed, I see black smoke burning its way up through my pelvis, and moving like a snake, it slithers up my spine.

I hear a scream that shocks me out of my meditation seat. I open my eyes and look around to find where the screaming is coming from. Zadie is by my side, her forehead wrinkled with concern.

"Lauren, are you okay?"

It was me. I was the one who screamed. Or was it that thing using my mouth to make noise? I shake my head "No" to Zadie's question and crawl towards the door. The black smoke is crowding me, filling me up. There isn't enough space for both of us. I need fresh air. I need open space. I need to get this thing out of me. It doesn't belong in me. We are not meant to be merged.

The chill of the night air greets me like a slap in the face. I can't see straight. I manage to stand up and lean over the porch railing for support. I am trembling so fiercely the earth begins shaking with me. Zadie and Gina follow me out.

"What happened?" Zadie asks.

Gina, my yoga teacher and mentor from home, comes and stands near me. With her familiar and steady gaze, I find my voice. "There is something inside of me!" I scream through tears.

"What?" Zadie asks.

"I don't know. It's dark and smoky and pushed its way out of my pelvis. It scared me!"

"Was it a rakshasa?" Gina asks.

"I think so. It felt like fire and like it was trying to push me out of my body. There wasn't room to breathe."

"Okay. Take a few deep breaths. Find your feet. Do you need to move a little?" Gina asks.

I nod and walk down the porch steps onto the paved driveway. I move up and down the driveway, taking small uneven steps. The trembling lessens and my breath begins to deepen and slow down.

"Lauren, is it still there?" Zadie asks.

I scan my body. I search through my spine and pelvis. I don't feel anything. "I don't think so. I can't feel it now if it is. That was really scary!"

"I think it's cool, Lauren!" Zadie laughs, her playful irreverence lightening the mood as always. "You always have the cool meditation experiences!"

I smile but don't laugh along with them all. Gina hands me my coat. I try to button it up but my hands are shaking too much. She sees my struggle and leans in to button it for me.

"Is everyone okay? We heard someone was upset!"

Paul's voice precedes him in the dark night. But then there he is, his face appearing above his lantern, taking us all in with his gaze. His eyes fall on me.

"It was me. I think I found a rakshasa in my pelvis. It scared me but I think it's gone."

"Mmmm . . . " Paul gazes at me intently. "It's not unusual for a rakshasa to appear after a lesson about them. They aren't able to hide anymore when you become aware of them. And your meditation practice is what then releases it: there is no room for that darkness in your growing light of consciousness."

I nod in response. His wisdom affirms what I realized yesterday: I am the one who can purify this energy. Me. The more consciousness and awareness I have, the less unconsciousness there is for these dark energies to lurk in.

I turn and follow Paul and the others to the dining hall for dinner. Is that the end? Is the rakshasa truly gone? Or is it waiting for me down in the depths of my meditative state? I reach down and put my hand on my pelvis. What else is down there waiting to emerge?

12

Me? Powerful?

PERU

I CAN'T BREATHE. I think I might throw up. What made me think I could do this? I look around the airport so quickly I get dizzy. The international terminal doesn't look different than the domestic side. I've traveled before but this is different. This time no one I know is waiting for me on the other side. The familiar red seats and chain restaurants I pass don't bring any comfort as I walk to the gate.

I concentrate on my breath as I move. My yoga training plays in my head—breathe through my nose, feel my feet on the floor, ground myself. This helps the spinning and I relax a little. I take a seat at Gate 38. I close my eyes and breathe in and out, in and out, in and out . . . until the world melts away.

A loud voice suddenly calls from the overhead speaker. Shit. She's speaking Spanish. We haven't even left the U.S. yet! I stand up quickly, surprising myself. I want to run. I want to leave. I want to go home and crawl into bed and forget about this adventure. Who needs to go to Peru to do yoga anyway? I do that here in Atlanta and have done just fine. Sure Peru has cooler mountains and hiking but I can do that here as well. Maybe I don't need to go. Maybe I'm not the adventuring kind . . .

I gather my things and turn to leave. I move away from the gate, away from the foreign language, away from the promise and fright of a new experience. As I walk away my eyes catch a flash of camouflage. Lean, tall, muscular bodies clad in army uniforms fill my sight. My heart races and I feel like I've been punched in the gut. David . . .

Flashes of the last few months shoot through my mind. Scenes from his funeral, his visits in my dreams, crying in the woods, wondering how he could die so young. Do I really want to keep running? What kind of life is that? I could die soon too. What would I have to show for it?

I remember the excitement I felt when I booked this trip. The fluttering in my stomach as I read about ten days of hiking, yoga with my favorite teacher and the resort's amazing healing gardens. The sense of accomplishment I had when I called Mom and Dad and told them that I was going—without having to check in with them first. At twenty-nine years old, it was the first time I had made a big decision on my own without consulting someone. This trip is for me.

I exhale with a huge whoosh. I didn't realize I had been holding my breath. I turn around to Gate 38 and see people lining up to board. I move forward and join the line. Step by step, breath by breath. I'm doing this. It's time to live.

THE WHISPERS RETURN

AS I GET OFF the plane my nose fills with pungent odors of soil, sweat and the open buckets people are using as toilets. I'm assaulted with loud Spanish that I can't understand and the squawk of chickens someone brought to the airport.

I see brown bodies wearing bright colored fabrics—reds, yellows and purples swirl in a moving rainbow in front of me. The humid air feels friendly, unlike the press of bodies pushing me forward and off the plane. I get jostled and prodded to the baggage claim. I see my blue suitcase that Mom and Dad gave me. The familiarity of the cool plastic handle feels good in my hands.

I look around and see a group of people standing with signs. A large one with

"Lauren Polly" written on it jumps out at me. Wow—that was easy. I breathe in deeply. My belly relaxes but my heart races as I approach the man with the sign.

"That's me," I say, pointing to the sign.

"Welcome Lauren Polly! Have a seat in the van. We'll leave soon." I follow to where his fingers point and enter the big white van. I'm relieved at the air conditioning and cushiony seats.

I stop abruptly at the sight of groups of two everywhere. Husband and wife, best girlfriends . . . I can feel the relationships and comfort between them immediately. I can also feel the borders around them. I'm on the outside. I smile shyly at the pairs of people as I make my way to the back of the van.

I knew there would be no one I knew waiting for me on the other end of the trip, but it doesn't stop the pit of loneliness in my belly from growing as I sit by myself and stare out the window.

Within minutes of sitting down I hear something. What is that? Whispers whoosh in my ears, filling my head with their echoing sounds of shhh and wshhhhh. They're familiar but I haven't heard them in years. I look around at my travel companions: do they hear this? No. Of course not. It's just my crazy returning. What's causing this?

More strangers have joined the group. More pairs of two are sitting in their invisible yet palpable bubbles with borders. Like Noah's Arc. There are a handful of people sitting on their own.

Some of them smile at me as I catch their eye. I turn my lips upward at them with an attempt at a smile and quickly turn my head to stare out the window. I feel like I'm fourteen again, being watched and hunted.

The whoosh in my ears and head grows. The whispers shiver down my spine. I feel them pushing at me from the inside out. The more they push, the tighter my skin feels. I run my fingers down my arms, imagining I'm cutting vents for the damn whispers to gush out. But it doesn't work. My belly wrestles with itself, churning and grinding. What's wrong with me? I try to breathe and center myself, but my meditation tricks aren't working here in Peru.

I look around at the people again. I get a few more smiles and some of them attempt to make small talk. Yet I can't hear them. Their voices are drowned out by the white noise of whispers. I smile politely and turn to stare out the window.

A deep voice from the seat beside me breaks through the whispers, "Lauren, tell me about your meditation practice."

"I'm studying with Paul. It's great. Just one mantra that you focus on. It's about not using effort or force."

"That must really be good for you."

His words stab me in the belly, *'That must be good for you.'* What is he talking about? What is he really saying? Why is it good for me? What's wrong with me that I need that? I smile politely at him and turn to look out the window.

"Have you ever been to Burning Man?" he asks, pulling me back. His attention is annoying.

"I've never heard of that before. What is it?" Why is he talking to me? Doesn't he see I want to be left alone?

"It's a festival for yoga, music. People check their inhibitions at the door and let themselves go. You should check it out. You'd be fun there."

I'd be fun? I feel like anything but fun. I feel pushy. I feel forced. I feel unnatural. And those damned whispers won't leave me alone. Why would anyone want me around? I squint at Peter. What's he up to? Is he like the kids in high school? Is he looking for my weak spots?

The van pulls to a stop at an old church. The trip leader calls out, "We're going to stop here and have a picnic lunch. Feel free to explore the grounds. The food will be in the back of the church when you are ready."

I give up my assessment of Peter as we all stand up to get off the van. I take the opportunity and flee from people. I feign interest in the trees so the few people who stop to chat with me leave me alone. As I stand with the trees, the whispers soften and quiet. Heat flushes up from my belly and brings with it a wicked voice:

I'm so pathetic. I'm so weak.
I don't fit in. I never did. I never will.
I don't want to be here anymore.

I wait for the others to pass, and then with a silent sob, I allow my tears to fall. Only the trees get to see my tears—no one else. What is happening to me? I haven't felt this way in years, not since I was in college.

I move slowly, breathing deeply as I do. There are more tears that want to come out but now isn't the time. I wipe my eyes and cheeks, locking the rest of the tears away as I head to the back of the church for lunch.

I take my bagged lunch and check out the options for seating. I cringe as flashes of the cafeteria at school come to mind. I move away from the crowd to sit on the foot of a statue of some saint. I breathe a bit more deeply and pick through my lunch. My belly surges in protest—it's too upset to digest anything.

"Lauren, that's a great spot!" One of the women exclaims. Her voice and genuine delight pull my attention up from my lunch. She is leading six people in my direction.

I smile but her openness and friendliness evoke more sadness. I scoot over to make room for them. As they sit down next to me I begin to feel pressed up against, even though they aren't touching me. My throat tightens. I desperately want space but I hold in my tears and breathe, smiling at them as they chat. I'm suffocating and no one can tell.

After lunch we return to the van and depart for the last short leg of the trip to the retreat center. I sit in silence and stare out the window. I hear a hissing sound, louder and more sinister than the whispers were. I curl my shoulders and move my head slightly, mimicking the slithering movements of a snake. I can feel my skin peeling away.

"Hey, can we stop here for photos?" someone calls out loudly. Photos? Stopping? What? I look out the window and take in the massive vista. Where was I? My breath catches in my throat as my heart bursts. It's so beautiful!

The van stops and we all clamber off to take photos. The group takes turns doing yoga poses on the cliff, snapping more photos of each other. I move away from them and stand at the cliff's edge, taking in the view that is larger and more open than anywhere I've ever been. The vibrant greens of the hills below pulse and glow. The jagged cliffs meld and sweep into softer curves. Bright yellow flowers dance in the wind. The rock pulses beneath my feet. These mountains are alive. I can actually feel my feet—and the mountain! The pulsing energy pushes its way up my feet. I begin to feel expansive inside, like when my inner world mirrored my outer world during my meditation retreat. I raise my face to the sky and close my eyes. For the first time all day my mind is quiet.

The wind picks up and twirls my hair. I lean into the sensual caress. The wind enters me but instead of soothing me as it usually does, it stirs me up. I open my eyes and stare down at the valley below. I hear the hiss again, louder and filled with contempt. *No one likes me. I don't like myself.* I can no longer see the beauty of the vista. I just see the gritty gray rocks hundreds of feet below me.

What would happen if I jump?

I pull myself away from the edge and walk quietly and quickly back to the van, where I stand and wait to be told it's time to board again. What was that? Something is wrong here. It's scaring me. I'm scaring myself.

It's Just Me Again

We arrive at the retreat center and are shown to our tents. I spend the rest of the day in silence. The hissing, the whispers, the thought of jumping . . . I am locked up inside myself again. There is a restorative yoga class being offered at sunset. I go.

I grab my mat, blankets and bolsters and take a spot in the back of the room. I can feel the yoga teacher, Desiree's wondering eyes on me. In her workshop back in Atlanta I was always front and center. I meet her gaze and she nods at me, understanding.

"We're going to do things a differently tonight. This is restorative yoga. We'll only do three or four poses and hold them a long time. I'll have some music on. Just get comfortable and relax."

She instructs us on how to use our bolsters to support our backs as we drape our bodies over them. I lay there, chest and legs open to the sky, feet together. I close my eyes. I feel so exposed and vulnerable in this pose. Tears spill out.

Desiree turns down the lights. The music is rhythmic. The female vocalist sings in a soft sensuous voice about the waves coming in and out. I feel the waves inside me build and swell. I can't hold it in anymore. I sob. The tears flow and make puddles on my bolster beneath my head. This time I don't hold any of it back.

Desiree comes and drops a tissue near my hand. I open my eyes and I smile at her in gratitude. Number one rule as a yoga teacher: if someone is crying in a release, don't touch or cuddle them. Hand them a tissue and let the release continue. The open space created for me to let go brings more waves of tears.

Eventually the sobs stop. The rhythmic music continues and I drop deep into the velvety stillness that is so soothing and healing to me. My breath opens and evens out. I tap into a deep peace. The hissing is gone. The whooshing is gone. The self-hatred is gone.

I'm just me again. Finally.

THE HEALER SPEAKS

IT'S DARK OUTSIDE AS I make my way back to the tent. I can't see the lush gardens but I can smell them. Roses: that's around the first bend, right? Orange blossoms—reminds me of Florida—that's around the second bend. I just need the lilies and then I turn right. It's Day 7 of the retreat and I'm starting to find my way around the grounds, even at night.

The glow from the fire in the tent greets me before the lilies do. The smell of smoke and incense take over the sweet smell of flowers. The smoke is heavy and coats my tongue as I crawl inside the tent.

Our tour guide, Lucita, greets me and says, "Lauren, this is Marisa, the Inca healer and psychic. I'll translate your reading for you if that's okay. I know it is private so be assured I won't talk to anyone about what is shared here."

"Okay," I reply, unable to take my eyes off the healer.

I smile and nod my head at Marisa as I take a seat on the floor across from both of them, sitting cross-legged like they are. I place my trembling hands on my thighs. I take a deep breath, wondering what's to come. The firelight dances in the corner of my vision; there's a strange glow around the small tent. I feel like I'm in a dream or have been sucked back in time.

I meet Marisa's brown eyes. As she looks deeply at me something stirs in my belly. She is scanning me the way the doctors used to but she seems to get in deeper. I fight the urge to shut her out. I relax, breathe and let her in.

Marisa moves quickly to her bag of cocoa leaves without talking. One of the other women at the retreat mentioned that this is how the healer "reads" you. She mutters some Spanish to Lucita.

"Pull out a handful of leaves and spread them on the ground in front of you," Lucita tells me.

I reach my hand into the brown burlap bag that Marisa holds out to me. My hand touches small, dry leaves. I gently take a handful and fan them out in front of me. I search the pattern curiously looking for what she might see in them.

Marisa looks at the pattern for a few moments in silence. My belly clenches and twists. I wipe sweat from my forehead. What will she see of my future? Oh no—what will she see of my past?

After a few minutes she smiles and raises her brown eyes to me, looking at me through the smoke. Her Spanish overlaps with Lucita's translation.

"You are special. You have gifts."

"No I don't."

Both women smile at my quick response. I tuck into myself, the way I used to at the shrink's office when receiving an assessment of myself. I get quiet and look for clues. What do they know about me that I don't know about myself?

"You have known great pain and struggle."

The clutching rises up from my belly and closes its hand around my heart. Oh no, she sees it. She sees it all.

"You think you are weak but you are stronger than most."

What?

"You have been afraid to show people your power. You need to stop that."

"I'm not powerful. What are you talking about?" My voice comes out rough and muffled as I choke back tears. What power?

"You are a clear channel of pure water. You have the ability to bring messages in from other times, other lands. You can teach the children. You can heal the earth."

I gasp. No. No, she doesn't see me at all. This is bullshit. I shake my head back and forth. I scratch at my arms.

"You are the rarest of people. We need you. The earth needs you to heal it."

Huge sobs push up from my belly and erupt. I shake and rock. The firelight and her words burn my skin.

Lucita squints at me. I can feel her walls going up around her so my sobs don't invade her space. I ache all over. I can feel her looking at me from behind her safe wall, assessing me like a wild animal caged for observation and entertainment. I sit on my hands to keep myself from clawing her.

Marisa sits calmly. Rather than pulling back like Lucita, she peers into me further. There are no walls around her. Her closeness is disturbing. Her placid face and soft eyes are pissing me off. She doesn't see. I have to make her see who I really am.

My voice rises over the sobs. "You don't understand. I'm sick. I'm crazy. I've been diagnosed with mental problems and on medication for years. I'm sick!"

"You are not sick or crazy! You are special. Powerful. Rare."

"But the doctors . . . "

"No."

"But for years I've . . . "

"No."

My protests fade in response to her certainty. She won't let me argue with her. As I look into her eyes all of me quiets. We sit in silence for several long moments. She continues on in a calm but commanding voice.

"You are a clear channel of water, but right now you are clogged with garbage. You need to purge to regain your power."

I nod in response.

"You need to know that you are safe. You are okay. Nothing bad will happen. It's time."

I feel a lightness in my belly. Is that hope?

"How do I purge?"

"You should always be dancing. It makes you happy, yes?"

I nod at her. She does see me.

"You should always be writing as well. There are untapped gifts there for you and for the world."

"Okay. I used to journal. The doctors had me do it as a way to release and reflect."

"Do it more. It will serve you well in the future to capture your words now."

I nod and enjoy the warmth of hope as it spreads from my belly and up my back.

I look over and into Lucita's observing eyes. She meets my gaze from behind her wall. She seems scared of me, and curious, too.

"Anything else?" I ask turning back to Marisa.

"Trust yourself. No one can do what you can do."

I uncross my legs and stand up. The fire warms my legs that are shaking under me. I turn away from the smoke, the firelight and the two Incan women. I leave the tent and am greeted by the stars. What does all this mean? Our conversation stays with me.

As I walk, as I journal, as I bend, twist and breathe on the yoga mat, as I sit silently at dinner tuning out the small talk, I hear her voice saying, "It is safe. You're okay. Nothing bad will happen. Trust yourself. You are special, rare, needed." Hope that what the healer said is true wrestles with the doubt and conviction that I'm sick and crazy. I don't have power. Do I?

In the dining room I catch Lucita looking over at me. I instinctively cower. She knows too much. She's too close. I'm not ready to be what was promised in the tent. I'm not sure if I ever will be. I smile politely at her; hiding whatever "power" they say I have from both of us.

MOON LIGHT RITUAL BATH

I TUG NERVOUSLY AT the strings of my bathrobe to make sure it is secure around my naked body as I follow Jose along the dirt path. We've left the paved trails behind us and are heading towards the woods. I follow the beam from his flashlight, walking cautiously on the uneven ground.

We enter the woods and he guides me to a small circular clearing. Steam rises from the tub set in the earth in the center of the meadow. The wind carries the heat of the steam towards us. The mix of cool and hot air caress my face and neck. The scent of lavender, rosemary and other unfamiliar herbs tickle my nose.

"Lauren, this is your bath. Stay as long as you like. The water is very hot: be careful. I'll leave this flashlight for you to find your way back when you are done." Jose smiles at me and slips back into the forest. I listen to his footsteps fade away and then there is silence except for the rustling of the trees. I'm alone.

I slip off my flip-flops and wiggle my feet in the soft grass that is still warm from the sun that set hours ago. I exhale loudly as I run my right foot lightly over the blades. The grass tickles my foot until I can't tell where one begins and one ends. I smile at the night sky. I can feel my feet again!

I slip out of my robe and stand naked in the moonlight. Closing my eyes, I feel the hot steam and cool night air stroke my body, changing directions with the wind. I moan with pleasure and surprise as the wind kisses my body again and again.

I see my old friends the stars twinkling and dancing. I allow the same dancing energy to come into the lightness in my belly. The familiar bubbles stir and build. They move up and out of me in soft giggles. I lift my arms overhead, letting myself get as big as the lightness inside.

I move to the bath. Large dark stones rim its edges. I see branches of herbs floating on the water but I can't see the bottom. It's both welcoming and mysterious.

I dip my big toe in to test the water and screech at the scalding temperature. I hop away and put my foot into the cool grass. It will be awhile before I can get in. I spread my bathrobe on the ground next to the tub and lie down on my back.

The right side of my body heats up at once with the steamy water right next to it. The left side is cool as the wind plays on my skin. I gaze at the twinkling stars beyond the swaying treetops. I melt into the earth.

The highs and lows of this trip have been exhausting. My fear of bipolar has been more in the forefront of my attention than it has since I was a teenager. I have gotten through it though. Like Marisa says—it's okay now. I'm safe.

The water eventually cools and I slide into the tub, moaning in delight as the tub accepts all of me. Only the top of my neck and head are exposed to the night air. I close my eyes as the warm water embraces my body.

Flashes of upset play behind my closed lids: the breakdown at the airport, the hissing and whooshing at lunch, the fear of my suicide contemplation at the edge of the cliff, the hate of myself that came in waves and was released with yoga . . . Flashes from my teen years play in the mix as well: the smoky snake, the cafeteria, the being hunted sensation at school, the pills I took to barter with God, my suicide letter. . .

But the pictures don't have the same impact anymore. The sting is softened and drowned out by the pleasure of the water and the sense of peace I feel. Marisa's eyes lit with firelight play last in this fast-moving picture show. Her deep, throaty Spanish and Lucita's translation play in my ears, "You are strong. Powerful. Rare." I almost believe her as I lie here in this decadent bath, with the stars sparkling down at me.

13

You Mean I'm Not Crazy?

IS IT TIME?

TODAY IS THE DAY. I step into the elevator and push the button for the 3rd floor. It's time. I know I'm ready. I'm going to talk with her about it. Will she agree? I spend the elevator ride breathing deeply to try and calm my jittery stomach.

The elevator doors open and I walk down the hall to Dr. S's office, which has become familiar to me now after coming to see her every three months for the past three years. She has seen me through my stressful days at Emory Hospital, my failed attempt at husband hunting and my new passion for yoga and meditation. During all this time I've been stable. I've been good; so good that I'm ready to make a big change.

"Hi Lauren," the secretary welcomes me. "You can go right in."

I knock softly on Dr. S's open door, "You ready for me?"

"Hi. Yes, come on in."

I enter and take my usual seat facing the window while silently greeting the magnolia trees. Dr. S moves to her chair carrying with her my chart and her yellow legal pad.

"So, how are you?"

I breathe in slowly, preparing to speak the words I've never spoken before. "I'm really good. I've been thinking that I would like to get off medication."

Dr. S looks up abruptly from her lap full of papers and pauses as she takes this in. "Okay. What brought this on?"

"It's been on my mind for a while now. As you know, typical bipolar needs to be managed with a heavy mood stabilizer and anti-depressants. I have been stable for seven years without an anti-depressant. And I'm not on a traditional mood stabilizer. I haven't been for ten years. The only drug I take now is Neurontin."

"That's true. And Neurontin is not even typically used for bipolar. Remind me, when were you started on that?"

As she flips through my chart I remind her of the details. "When I was eighteen and leaving for college. I saw a specialist in Baltimore who recommended it. Originally I was taking 900mg. My current dosage is written for 300mg and I usually forget the middle of the day dose. I've only been taking 200mg for the past few years with no trouble. I've noticed that most of the patients that I work with in the hospital are on 900mg or higher... My dosage seems sub-clinical to be effective. Maybe I don't need it at all."

"Well, you have been on medicine for over half of your life. Since fourteen and you are now thirty. So we would need to work slowly and titrate you down to get totally off it. You wouldn't want to just stop abruptly. And I'll want to follow you more closely."

"I understand that. I'm willing to do whatever you need. I want to give it a try."

"You are still doing yoga and meditating? Eating well? Sleeping patterns are normal and regulated?"

"Yes. I think I can manage myself that way."

Dr. S pauses and stares at me for a few moments. "Yes. I think so, too. Okay. We will titrate the dosage down slowly and gradually over the next few months. We'll go down in 50mg increments. I want you to be on top of this. If anything pops up you call immediately."

I let out a sigh of relief. I'm ready. I knew it. Dr. S writes a new prescription for 50mg pills. We smile at each other as I take the paper from her. This is it! This may be the last prescription I ever get.

THE PAYOFF

I MAKE MY WAY through the full studio to the front of the class. I take a big breath as I turn and face them all. There are about forty people here for my class. Forty! I usually teach to smaller groups at another studio across town. I'm the guest teacher tonight in a new yoga studio. The room is buzzing with conversations.

I take another deep breath and speak, "Good evening and happy Sunday everyone! I'm Lauren and I'll be leading class today. Thank you all for coming." I smile into the sea of unfamiliar faces.

"Please take a cross-legged position as we take a minute to set the intention and theme for today's practice." I pause as people find their way to their mats. As I watch them move I note whose back is stiff, who is moving with ease and who is connected to their body. I breathe deeply to calm the nervous butterflies in my stomach.

"I know that as we near Thanksgiving, most teachers are talking about being grateful. I sense you've had your fill of that!" I smile at them and get many smiles and heads nodding in return.

"So tonight we're going to work on staying grounded and open during the stress of the holidays. How often do you get overwhelmed during the busiest, most stressful, family drama time of the year? How often do you start pushing your way through what you need to do instead of checking in with your body, your health and well-being?" I pause and look around the room as more heads nod.

"With yoga we learn to use the breath, be present and soften into the moment. We open to grace and stop efforting as much. We then are able to find our feet, so to speak, to allow us to hold steady during times of stress. This is what we'll be focusing on tonight with and through our bodies. Please close your eyes and join me with three OMs."

I feel the excitement of exploring these bodies and how to guide them into more fluidity take over. The nervous jitters settle. My instruction and movement come easily. The sea of bodies swell and dive, ebb and flow throughout the next ninety minutes.

My voice leads the way and the bodies follow. Leaving space between the words allows the minds to get quiet and present. My succinct directions of the poses give clarity on how to move the body. Intermittent messages of opening, softening into the breath and feeling the feet carry the simple movements into life lessons, something for people to keep with them when they leave.

"Before you begin to move, soften first. Open to something bigger and see if that stops your push."

"Feel your feet on the ground, hold yourself steady in the pose. And can you remain soft at the same time?"

"Balance and find steadiness inside of you. How can you use this as you move through the stress of the holidays?"

"Take time to be here. Don't let your mind go to other people. Be present for yourself."

We end in a savasana. This is the usual closing pose for all classes. I guide everyone to lie down on their backs with their arms by their sides. I sit at the front of the room and survey the group. The sweat on the foreheads, the small smiles playing on a few lips, the deepened breath, the relaxation after movement. I watch as the collective breath stills, the silence grows and the relaxation deepens. I close my eyes, melting into meditation, taking the group into a deeper space with me.

A gentle chime rings to mark the end of the session. I bring myself up from meditation and pause before speaking, savoring the silence.

"Slowly wiggle your fingers and toes, coming back into presence with your body. Roll onto your right side and slowly make your way to a seat." I pause as the bodies are brought back to the same pose we started with, completing the cycle.

"Remember, as you are moving about the busyness of life, in particular this holiday season, to take time for you. Soften, relax, open up and find your feet in the midst of the stress and drama. Find your steadiness and you can handle anything."

I place my hands in prayer position in front of my chest and bow my head, saying, "Namaste." The silence of the class is interrupted with loud clapping and cheering. I look up quickly in surprise. I'm used to a quiet, group "Namaste," in response; not this.

"Thank you?" I say, laughing softly.

I look around the room to the calmer, happier, more present people. I take in the more fluid relaxed bodies. This is the payoff from all my naked yoga. I *can* guide people on how to enter their own bodies, and I realize I'm pretty good at it. I stand up and am greeted by one happy body after another, wishing to give me a hug of appreciation.

I Don't Belong in a Box

"How's it going?" Dr. S asks me.

"I'm fine," I say, laughing softly. She smiles in return.

"You've been off meds for four months now. No problems?"

"No problems." I smile at her, basking her in the glow of how happy I am to report this.

"Okay. Congratulations! At this point you are good to go. I would like to follow you every six months just to check in as needed. And if anything occurs—any mood swings—call me immediately."

I nod reassuringly, "I know. I will." I pause before asking this next question. I've been giving this a lot of thought. "Do you think I was ever really bipolar? I don't seem to fit into that category now. I'm not sure I did back then either." Memories of my research in the library flash through my mind. I remember how I saw this as learning a new character role.

"Well, you have to remember that that was over half your lifetime ago. Who's to say? I would ask now if it really matters."

"I guess not. What do you think was wrong with me?"

"From what I see now I would say you are not bipolar. I would say you have a tendency towards severe depression and anxiety and that you manage yourself beautifully with all of your stress techniques, yoga and life style."

"So . . . I'm not bipolar?"

Dr. S meets my eyes and says without hesitation, "No. I would say you are not bipolar. Which leads me to a quandary: what do I put on your billing form?"

I laugh at her directness. I know the billing forms all too well from the hospital. You need a diagnosis to bill insurance. You need a box to put people in to prove that what you did helped them.

"What box do I belong in now?" I tease.

Dr. S stares at the paper and sighs. "I'm just going to check this one."

I stand to peer over her shoulder and see a tiny black check mark next to "Unspecified mood disorder."

"Interesting choice. But I don't think I belong in any box."

"None of us do, Lauren. None of us do."

YOU ARE A VERY POWERFUL WOMAN

I MELT INTO THE massage table as Brian, an energy and structural body worker, taps his fingers along my back and down my legs. My new chiropractor in San Francisco recommended I come see Brian to work on my adrenals, which are fatigued from living in a fight-or-flight state all the time. I'm glad I came. The tightness in my hips and pain in my neck are now gone. My breathing is calmer.

Brian moves to my feet and applies pressure. Acupuncture points? I wonder. I feel a rush of energy up my back as my spine adjusts itself like magic. I exhale loudly. I can sense when Brian lifts his hands off my feet and sits down in his chair a few feet away. I linger on the table, savoring the softness of my body.

I open my eyes, adjusting to the golden light in the room. I slowly roll to my side and sit up, meeting Brian's eyes. "Thank you, Brian. I feel amazing." My voice sounds different to me. It's slower, deeper.

"You are so welcome. You are interesting to work on. You are very different."

I feel a flutter in my chest. What does he mean? He sees the question in my eyes. "Your spirit guided me throughout the treatment, showing me specifically how to work on your body to help you get the most from this healing."

What is he talking about? "No one has ever said something like this to me before. Do you experience things like this with other clients?"

"Yes and no. I have never had that much clear communication from a spirit about their body before. And certainly not in my first session with someone." He pauses and takes a deep breath before continuing, "You are a very powerful woman, Lauren."

I stare at his blue eyes that are now sparkling in excitement, like a child who has found a hidden gem. The glow from the lamp on his desk makes me think of the firelight during my reading from the healer in Peru.

"I had a session with a healer in Peru a few years ago. She said something similar. She said I was powerful, and rare also."

Brian smiles. "The rarest. You are one who was brought back to earth to change the world." I hear his words and doubt rises in my mind. It seems so big. How can I do that?

"That's what she said, too. But I wasn't willing to consider what she told me. I kind of shut it out. It seemed so, so . . . lofty."

"It is lofty, but so are you. You aren't quite human."

What? For a moment I can't breathe. What the hell am I then?

Brian laughs softly. "It's okay. To me you are much more angel than human. A super powerful one. I can't wait to see what you will create in this world. I'm happy I get to work with you."

His genuine gratitude and kindness flow to me like a warm gentle wave and I take a deep breath. Flashes of the Peruvian translator come quickly to mind: her assessing eyes; her look of curiosity mixed with fear; the way she seemed to put up invisible walls between us.

I look at Brian: no assessment, no fear, no walls, just curiosity. What would it be like to have that for myself? No fear, just curiosity?

"I've been afraid of being different, being powerful. Especially after my mental issues. I was told that was the mania. Grandiose ideas and all of that."

"What if it's something different?"

"Yes. What if . . . "

I sit for another few moments in silence before standing up to put on my shoes. "I'm starting work with the energy psychologist next door, Dr. P, next week. Maybe it's time I look at this."

"That sounds like an excellent start."

YOU'RE NOT CRAZY—YOU'RE REMEMBERING

MY BELLY FLUTTERS. I wonder what we're going to explore today? As I sit in Dr. P's waiting room I remember my hesitation at seeing a therapist again, but my chiropractor suggested I come. My neck adjustments aren't holding and she thinks it's because of unresolved emotional issues.

So I consent to go and quickly discover that Dr. P and her "Energy Psychology" are very different from the talk therapy I did for years. I don't run circles in my mind anymore. Instead, something very different happens here.

My reflection is interrupted as Dr. P opens her office door, "Lauren, I'm ready for you." Her red curls bounce as she turns around, inviting me to follow. I smile as I enter her office. Between the orange leather couch and shag rug I feel like I've stepped back into the '70s.

"How's it going?" Dr. P asks.

"Okay. I've been thinking a lot about my need to stay hidden. I always thought this came from having a bipolar diagnosis. I didn't want people to know I was crazy. I thought if I hid I would be safer from judgment. I'm really ready to change this. I don't want to stay hidden. Can we clear this?"

"Of course we can. Let's start with some NET and go from there."

Dr. P uses a variety of different tools in our work together. NET (Neuro Emotional Technique) uses muscle testing to tap into my body's knowledge. It helps us identify—and release—the emotions I'm holding in my body, from the past decades and even from past lifetimes!

This approach is a real stretch for me: past lives? I had learned about reincarnation in yoga and even though this is weird, I'm seeing shifts already in our short time together. My mind is more relaxed and I'm discovering that my body is really wise.

Dr. P also uses tools from Access Consciousness™. In our first session together she introduced me to something called the "Light/Heavy Tool." She asked me questions and then invited me to tune into the energy in my body and in the space around me: did I feel light or heavy? A "light" sensation is a 'yes' or a truth for me. A "heavy" sensation is a 'no' or an un-truth.

After decades of seeing doctors who claimed to know more than me and told me what was going on with my body, I'm now learning how to listen to what my body and I know. I'm being asked the questions. I'm the one finding out what is true for me. I'm becoming my own expert on me.

Dr. P sits next to me and invites me to hold my arm out straight. Using the NET technique she alternates between asking questions and gently pressing down on my arm. My arm either stays in place or it falls down. This is the NET version of the Light and Heavy tool.

"So repeat after me, 'It's safe for me to be seen.'" I repeat this statement and she pushes gently down on my arm. My arm falls.

She asks more questions and we discover that all of this is connected to a past life where it wasn't safe for me to be seen.

"So what comes up for you? What are you aware of?" Dr. P asks.

"Mmm...," I pause. I have a sense of something, but it's not from this lifetime. How could that be? Am I making it up? I share with her what I'm aware of, "It feels like I was killed or sent away when I was seen."

"Okay," Dr. P nods, as though all of this is very normal and not make-believe. "Were you doing something or being something you weren't supposed to?"

I smile at the answer that pops in my head. Do I dare say this out loud? "I was a witch. Or at least they thought I was one."

"And what happened?"

"I was sent away."

"So what happens when you are seen?"

"I get ostracized and sent away."

We sit in silence for a moment, looking at each other. Then Dr. P continues with asking questions, testing my arm strength, and touching specific points on my body that help release the blocked emotion and memories from this past lifetime.

We continue on for a while and then she has me say again, "It's safe to be seen." This time when I repeat the statement my arm stays strong. Finally, I'm willing to be seen. No more hiding. No more being blocked by this past lifetime.

"How do you feel?"

"Good. Lighter. It's still strange for me to talk like this: about past lifetimes and being aware of different energies, like we talked about last time. But so much of what we talk about is also so familiar..." I pause as I realize how all that we have talked about is so "light" and true for me.

"But every time I told the doctors about these things—the whispers and the wind and even that experience with the thunderstorm I told you about—they told me it was all part of my craziness."

Dr. P looks right into my eyes and says, "Lauren, you weren't crazy. You were remembering. There's a difference."

I stop breathing; the certainty of her words grab my breath away. I wasn't crazy. I was remembering. This feels light to me.

"So I was remembering?"

"Yes. You were—and are—remembering the gifts you had from past lifetimes. You once knew how to communicate with these energies and 'whispers'. You once knew that communion with the trees and land around you was natural, instinctual. You once had capacities—or skills—for hearing the truth of what was going on for someone beyond the words they said. The mismatch between those—the words and energies—probably had you feel crazy in this lifetime!"

I nod.

"You weren't crazy though. You never were. You were remembering all these gifts you had but you didn't have any way of knowing how to use them. It's like you were a sculptor with all these blocks of clay—all this raw material—but you had no tools to shape it or work with it."

"Wow," I whisper. This is so different from what any of the other doctors has ever told me. Yet it feels so light.

"I'd like to learn more. I kind of want to go and get a book about witches."

"There are bookstores full of this stuff, especially in San Francisco. I say go for it, Lauren. No one hunts witches anymore. No one will come and take you away. It is safe for you to explore. It is safe to be seen, remember? Why don't you go check out some books and see what you find out?"

I float out of her office, knowing exactly where I'm going next. With her permission, I'm going to explore.

14

Reclaiming All of Me

EXPLORATION

THE CRYSTALS IN THE store window twirl in slow circles, sparkling in the sunlight and offering out rainbows in return. I glance up at the sign above the door: "Angel Bookstore," it says in big purple letters.

The letters seem to swim on the sign. I blink a few times. I look again. The words have stopped swimming. I take a deep breath and put a hand on my belly. I'm just exploring, I remind myself. I'm just exploring. I push open the door and hear a chime. I freeze in the doorway: I feel like a child who has been caught with my hand in the cookie jar.

"Welcome!" a dark-haired woman says to me from the counter. "Are you here for the workshop?"

What workshop? I swallow, trying to get rid of a sudden lump in my throat. I still can't move from the doorway.

I hear Dr. P's voice in my ear, *"No one hunts witches anymore. No one will come and take you away. It is safe for you to explore."* I take a deep breath and walk into the bookshop, letting the door close behind me.

"I was just coming to look at books. I didn't know there was a workshop."

"We just started a few minutes ago. It's not too late to join."

I feel a flutter in my chest. "What's it about?"

"The healing power of stones and crystals."

The fluttering quickly turns into pounding. All of a sudden I feel hot. I swallow again, noticing there's still a lump in my throat. Crystals. . . do I dare? Now it's my mother's voice that rings in my ear, *"All those depressing books you were reading and the crystals you were playing with...that's what brought on the darkness."*

I surprise myself as the words, "Yes, I'd like to do it," tumble out of my mouth.

"Great! They are gathered in the room just down that hallway," she says, pointing to the other side of the store. "Just head in and have a seat."

Before I know it, I'm walking across the store, down the hallway and entering the workshop. The speaker smiles at me and keeps talking to the group of women sitting around a table. I take the closest seat to the door, trying to be as quiet as I can. Is it okay for me to be here? And then I catch myself. *"It's safe to be seen."* Right. I'm okay.

There are stones and crystals of different colors and shapes laid out on a cloth on the table. They are organized in groups by color, creating a rainbow of sorts. I look around at the other people. Two look like housewives and two are my age. They don't look weird. They look normal.

I look up at the speaker. I realize how familiar this feels: there is a teacher and there are students. Just like in my graduate school classes and yoga. My shoulders drop down from where they were hanging out by my ears. I am exploring. I am a student.

"The stones work well with chakras, too, if you know what those are." I smile and nod. Chakras, once foreign, are now familiar to me. I give Dr. T a silent thank you.

"I invite you to hold the stones and see what you feel and notice with each one." More permission to explore.

I hold a dark black stone in my hand and notice the bottom of my feet buzzing.

The bright orange stone ignites a small fire in my belly. The pink crystal makes me smile. I hold it up to my chest and close my eyes. I notice a little fluttering sensation in my heart, like butterflies. We each have a chance to describe our experience. I smile and laugh with the other women as they describe similar sensations to what I was noticing. At the end of the workshop we all clap as the speaker thanks us for coming. I slide out of my chair and head back out into the bookstore. As I walk by the counter I feel a shiver up my spine and a tug at my attention. I look over and gasp as a familiar dark gray smoky crystal grabs my gaze.

I move quickly over to the glass case that houses the more expensive stones. The gray beauty is sitting in the middle of the display amidst pure clear quartz stones. The contrast of the smoky darkness in a sea of clarity is breathtaking.

"Do you know about smoky quartz?" the speaker asks, coming up behind me.

"I had a necklace with one when I was in middle school. It's used for protection and defense, right?"

"Yes and so much more than that. Smoky quartz transforms negative energy of any kind to positive energy." Well, that would be helpful with dealing with the hospital stress, I think to myself.

"It is a stone that brings abundance, prosperity, and good luck." Who wouldn't want that?

"Emotionally, smoky quartz is excellent for elevating moods, overcoming negative emotions and relieving depression. It is very calming and is considered a serenity stone."

Hmmm . . . it didn't help me with that when I was younger. A memory flashes through me of the day I stood in the corner of my room, cowering, feeling a presence watching me. Was it coming from the crystal? I never knew. After that day I never wore the crystal again. What if it could be different now?

"Let me open the case and you can hold it." She inserts a big brass key into the lock. The clicking of the lock is loud and cuts through the buzz in my head from the memory. She takes out the smooth gray stone carved like a pyramid and hands it to me.

The stone is cool to the touch. My feet buzz like they did with the other black stone during the workshop. I take in a deep breath and notice my neck and shoulders soften and feel more fluid.

I hold the crystal up to the light and see darker shades of gray and brown streaks, like wispy clouds streaking the sky. The light bounces off the streaks with a rainbow of colors just like the crystals in the window. It's beautiful. I don't feel sucked into it like I did with the smoky quartz I had as a teenager. This is different. I want to explore it more. It feels soothing, not dangerous.

I surprise myself yet again as I say, "I'll take this one."

"Good choice," she says. "You can keep looking around if you like and I'll wrap it up and have it waiting for you on the counter when you're ready to pay."

She takes the crystal with her to the counter and I start to move towards the books: my path is blocked by one of the younger women from the workshop. Her bright blue eyes are lined in heavy black eye liner and mascara. They are in such contrast to her fair skin and blonde hair, kind of like the smoky quartz surrounded by clear quartz in the case.

"Are you going to get it?"

"Yes. It's beautiful!"

"It is. Hi. I'm Kelly. Is this your first workshop here?"

"I'm Lauren. Yeah, I was just coming to browse the books. I was interested in reading up on witches and ghosts." Did I really just tell her that?

"Oh! I have a ghost in my apartment right now. That's how I found this place. I was trying to find out how to get rid of it."

My heart pounds and there is a ringing in my ears. She has a ghost? Did it come here with her? I shiver as goose bumps appear on my arms. I take a step back. But my curiosity gets the best of me. "How do you know you have a ghost?"

"I get shivers. Sometimes I see things move. I even felt him crawl into bed with me a few times. That was really creepy." I feel like I might throw up at the thought of sharing my bed with a ghost.

"How about you? Have you ever felt them?" Have I? Is it safe to share with this stranger?

"Well, I used to hear whispers when I was younger. Sometimes it seemed like something was pulling me to move in a certain direction. I just thought I was crazy."

"Yeah, I thought that too at first until I started reading up on it. It seems a lot of people have encounters with ghosts. I just want this one to get out of my house. He feels creepy. I bought a bunch of black tourmaline jewelry to wear which makes me feel better. It's supposed to protect you. I wear it at work too."

"Where do you work?"

"I teach third grade."

I take a small step forward. Third grade? That's so . . . sweet. And normal. She smiles at me and I smile back.

"Well, maybe I'll see you at their next workshop."

"Yeah, maybe," I say. "Good luck with getting rid of your ghost."

She heads over to one section of books and, wondering where I would find books on witches, I head on impulse down the row closest to me and stop as I see the "Witches" label right above me. My chest thumps. I look around to see if anyone is watching me. Nope. I move forward and read the titles. A book with a photo of a bright green forest catches my eye. As I reach to pick it up I hear a noise behind me. I pull my hand back quickly and look around.

It's another woman checking out books, too. She smiles at me. "That one you were reaching for is good. It's about nature magic and how you can harness the energy in the earth."

"Oh, thanks," I say and reach back to pick up the book. She isn't coming to get me. She isn't judging me. She's looking at the same section of books that I am!

I flip through the book and see that it's divided into sections based on the five elements. The five elements. Hmmm. Like what I learned in my yoga teacher training and that I now teach to others: how to be more in tune and embody each element: earth, air, fire, water and space.

Guiding my yoga students to feel their connection to the five elements is so natural to me and it always seemed helpful for them. Dr. P's voice rings in my ears again, *"There is no harm in exploring."* I carry the book with me to the cash register where my crystal is waiting.

THE BOOK COMES ALIVE AGAIN

THE FIVE ELEMENTS. YOGA. Chakras. Earth, air, fire, water, space . . . Everything I learned from Dr. T and my yoga teachers floods through me as I sit at home with my new book in my lap. It's as though by purchasing the book I'm activating all the knowledge I have on these related topics. Is that how it works? Is it activating my past life as a witch, too?

I gaze into my smoky crystal sitting on the table beside me. I remember one of the first yoga classes I taught. I guided the students through specific balancing postures to embody the earth element. Through these postures we strengthened our foundation to feel more grounded and secure. Will this Natural Magic book be like this, too? Filled with practical, helpful information?

I look down at the glossy cover and the light from the lamp reflects off it, shining in my eyes. I close my eyes and take a deep breath, asking the pounding in my chest to settle down. "There is no harm in exploring," I whisper to myself.

I flip through the chapters about the five elements and how to work with them. A lot of what the author explains matches up with what I've already learned from yoga. I skip ahead, seeking new information.

Words jump off the page at me mid-way through the book: *how to use the power of the wind to turn things your way.* What? Use the power of the wind to turn things my way? What is she talking about?

I gaze back at my smoky quartz as goose bumps spread up my arms. I love feeling the wind caress my skin, play with my hair and move through me. That gentle communion with the wind seems so innocent. But then I remember my standoff with God and the thunderstorm. The wind picking up, responding to my anger; the rolls of thunder and bolts of lightning . . .

I shiver as I realize what might have happened had things turned out my way during that storm. Would I want to use the power of the wind to turn things my way? What does that actually mean? Control the wind?

I flip forward a few pages and another sentence leaps off the page: *how to control a person's thoughts.* What is this? This is so strange. Using earth magic to control others? More goose bumps cause me to shiver, as the words seem to pulse and creep out of the book into my fingers and up my arms.

I don't want to use magic to control others. That's not what I'm interested in. What kind of magic am I interested in? I don't even know, really... I'm just exploring. What am I looking for? I want to know how to use my gifts. If I was once a witch, what kind of magic did I know? What did I use it for?

I'd like to be able to talk to those energies that come and visit me. I'd like to communicate with the wind and the whispers. I'd like to know what they are saying. I'd like to learn their language: the language of the earth and the elements. That's what I want.

Another phrase grabs my attention: *you can set up an altar and hold rituals daily.* A collage of images and memories bombard me. The image of my altar that I sit at during meditation. It has two statues: Shiva and Green Tara. I have my prayer beads on it and things that I collect while out on my walks, like pretty leaves and stones. I learned about having this kind of altar from Paul. He encourages all his students to create a space that focuses our attention and our mind during our sitting practice. So how is this different?

Memories of my youth flash in my mind: dipping my smoky crystal in salt to purify it—and me. Putting salt in bowls in my room to purify the space. My mom's voice, *"All those depressing books you were reading and the crystals you were playing with . . . that's what brought on the darkness."*

What would it be like to play with these energies on my own, without a teacher? What would I remember from when I was a witch? The pulsing continues to move up my arms and into my chest around my heart. I can't catch my breath.

This feels wrong. This feels heavy in my body. An invisible hand squeezes my heart as the pulsation continues to move down into my belly. No. No. I won't play with these energies. I don't want the darkness. I throw the book across the room and stand up, shaking my body to release that pulsing energy. "Get out," I command.

I reach my arms overhead and stretch, inhaling I lean to the left, exhaling I lean to the right, just like in my yoga classes. Inhale, exhale. I do this over and over again until the heavy hand around my heart loosens its grip.

GHOSTS

"CAN WE TALK ABOUT the presences?" I shift from side to side on Dr. P's couch. My hands, like my belly, are clenched in balls.

"Sure."

"When I was younger I felt like someone was there with me, watching me, but there wasn't anybody physically there. And sometimes I heard whispers. Lots of whispers. I heard them at school and when I was alone . . . " I trail off. How do I talk about this?

Dr. P leans her head to the side and asks me bluntly, "So are you aware of ghosts?"

I start to shake my head. Of course I'm not aware of ghosts. That would be creepy and weird. I can't even watch horror movies without being freaked out for weeks. Yet as she asks me the question I feel a lightness in my body and in the space around me and remember what this is telling me; it's telling me this is a truth for me.

"It's light for me, so . . . yes." We've been using more of the Access Consciousness tools lately. Dr. P says she's seeing quicker results with her clients with these tools.

"Is that okay with you?" she grins at me.

"I'm scared of them. I could always feel something there but it's like, I didn't *want* to see it."

"Are you scared of people in bodies?"

"Well, no."

"Why would you be scared of people without bodies?"

Good point. But . . . "Sometimes they feel so invasive. So pushy. When I was going crazy it was intense, like whooshing inside my head. And one time I was with my family in Savannah and it got really intense. I felt like they were tugging at me to follow them to the cemetery. What did they want from me?"

"So were they trying to get your attention?"

"That's light, so yes."

"Is there someone now trying to get your attention?"

I sit and pay attention to the space around me and inside of me. I notice a slight pushing energy on my right and a lot of lightness inside. I look into the empty space and see nothing but I know it's there.

"There is someone here."

Dr. P nods. "Who is it?"

Without hesitation I share what I am immediately aware of, "My father from another life."

"What does he want?"

I get quiet and listen. At first I don't hear or notice anything. That's when I become aware of a thick energy around me. I close my eyes and ask myself, "What is this?" I realize it's a wall of protection I've put up around me energetically.

I take a deep breath and on my exhale imagine I'm pushing the walls down with my hands. I'm not scared of people in bodies so why should I be scared of him? I am instantly flooded with an energy of concern. I blink back tears.

"He's worried about me. He wants to know if I'm okay."

"Are you okay?"

"Yes."

"Good. Can you tell him that and see if that lets him leave?"

I pause and get still. The wall comes up again as I tune into him. I push it down. "I'm okay," I tell him. "I'm okay, you can go." His presence with its slight push begins to dissipate.

"He's going now."

"Is he gone completely or do we need to clear him to help him go?"

"What's a clearing?"

"You know how in your meditation you focused on 'dipping into the fire' as you called it and burning away the unconsciousness so you could be pure light?"

"Yes."

"Well, it's kind of like that for these energies that I call entities and others call ghosts. Sometimes these entities get stuck here and don't realize they can leave this reality. They're, well, you could say they are anxious and are asking for help to change that. So when we 'clear' them, we burn away the unconsciousness and help them feel more at peace. Usually when we do this they leave you alone, too."

I ask myself, does he need a clearing? That feels light in my body. "Yes. He needs a clearing."

Dr. P says what she calls the special entity clearings. The space around me changes as she says it. His presence gets lighter and lighter and then he is gone. I don't feel him there anymore. I notice that my fists and belly are no longer clenched.

"That wasn't so scary was it?" Dr. P asks.

"Well, no. It wasn't scary. It felt peaceful once I was able to get my walls to drop down and tune into him."

"It just takes practice. You'll get more comfortable with it. And the next time you feel a presence—or hear the whispers—know it's an entity. You can ask it questions. You can do this by yourself whenever you want to."

I smile back at her. From bipolar diagnosis to communicating with the entities. Some people might still call me crazy but that matters to me less and less. I like this kind of exploration. I like the freedom. I like being my own expert.

As I leave Dr. P's office, she asks, "What else is possible?"

Indeed! What else is possible? I wasn't crazy, I was remembering. I wasn't hallucinating, I'm aware of ghosts. What other psychological problems did I have in the eyes of the doctors that were actually gifts that I have?

THE (PAST-LIFE) WALK

DEEP EMERALD GREENS SURROUND ME. They are so rich in color they seem to vibrate. After hiking fast up the hill, my face is sweaty and it feels good to slow down and breathe in the beauty of the forest.

Florescent green curly moss calls out to me to touch it from where it's perched on the side of a pine tree. It tickles as I run my hand over it. I can feel the aliveness of the tree trunk the same way I would feel a person beneath their patch of hair.

I look up high into the branches and smile at the tree in greeting. It sways in the breeze as if waving hello to me. Sunlight streaks down through the branches, bathing my face in warm kisses.

I look down to explore the moss. Its curls sparkle in the sunlight. It winds its ways around the trunk and down to the ground beneath. Its bright color is even more striking against the earth, darkened from the recent rain. I breathe in deep to smell the slight must of wet earth. I can almost taste the moisture that remains in the air.

I sit in the tree's lap made by a few unearthed roots. I rest into the tree, adjusting a bit till I find a position where the roots support me, rather than jab at my back.

I untie my hiking boots and peel off my thick socks. My toes wiggle wildly with joy at being unbound and caressed by the cool air. A bubble of pleasure builds in my pelvis and rises up and out in a laugh.

I sink my toes into the ground and the smell of moss and earth fills me up. I sink back into the tree and close my eyes, allowing this smell of home to carry me back in time. Scenes of my parents barefoot, covered in dirt and laughing with each other as they tend to the flowers, flow through my mind.

The picture of my parents fades as I drop deeper. I go through the velvet blackness so familiar to me now with meditation. More pictures arise. I see dirty feet and firelight. They are not familiar images and I sense they are memories from some distant time.

I open my eyes and see the empty hiking trail. The dirt path twists and turns between trees and shrubs. It is a maze of green and brown, well worn with time and other travelers. As I stare at the trail it starts to wiggle and all the colors swim in front of my eyes the way the letters did on the bookstore sign. A simultaneous picture flashes of another trail that looks very similar. I have been there before. I have been here before. I am in both places. My heart pounds with a strange recognition. I shake my head to clear the double vision and swimming pictures.

My sessions with Dr. P come to mind. We have been exploring my past lives, discovering all these different versions and stories of myself: the witchy woman, the warrior, the sword dancer. As I remember these past lives I reclaim the gifts and capacities I once had.

"You're not crazy. You're just remembering." Dr. P's reassuring words flow through me. *"You're not crazy. You're just remembering."*

As I look at the winding trail I sense all these different versions of me here, waiting, watching, remembering with me. I stand slowly and begin to walk down the path barefoot. With each step I ask the earth to show me: show me me. I ask all of those versions of me that I have recently discovered, as well as all of those yet to be discovered, to come and play. I ask them to join with me. I am ready to reclaim all of me.

As I move down the trail I see images from my adolescence mixed with my past lives:

> *Battling with a smoky snake by my side.*
> *Being the warrior leader in ancient China.*
>
> *Facing off with God during the thunderstorm.*
> *Being the wizard who played with the elements of the earth.*
>
> *Sword dancing in my parents' bedroom.*
> *Being a sword dancer in Spain.*
>
> *Hearing the whispers in the wind.*
> *Being the witch who communicated with spirits.*
>
> *Fear of my power.*
> *Being the one who was ostracized and killed for being different.*

With each image I feel a sense of recognition and instantly the energy of the past me flows into my body. All of those strengths that I had once made myself wrong for, or refused, were capacities. Gifts. As I walk barefoot down the trail I am joined by all of me, from this lifetime and past lifetimes.

I'm vibrating head to toe. I'm expanding in every possible direction. The more pictures I see the larger I get. The more energy comes. I am not fragile. I am not brittle. I am not "poor little Lauren." I am filling up with the power of me.

Dr. P's voice rings in my mind, *"Your light shines so bright it would blind others. What better gift to the world?"* Bubbles explode in my pelvis and rise through me in waves of laughter. I expand as more light, more laughter, more of me.

I am barefoot and free. Freer than I have been in a long time. Maybe more free than I have ever been. I recall the tool Dr. P shared with me: ask a question for more to show up.

I smile and ask out loud, "How does it get better than this?"

IS IT MINE? OR SOMEONE ELSE'S?

"THERE IS SO MUCH yuck at work."

"Well, Lauren. You do work in a hospital," Dr. P shrugs her shoulders and smiles at me. Her red curls bounce, emphasizing her point.

"I know. It's hard. I feel sad all the time."

"Is it yours?"

"What do you mean, is it mine?"

"Is that sadness yours or are you aware of everyone else's sadness?"

"Um, you lost me . . . "

"So this is another Access Consciousness tool that I use myself and with my clients. Just like some of the other tools I've shared with you, it may sound weird at first. Are you interested in trying it to see what you might discover?"

I look at her framed diplomas on the wall behind her head. The tools she shares with me are so different, just like she is so different. Just like Dr. T was so different. Yet it works. We clear stuff quickly rather than needing to talk about issues for months and months as I did with the therapists. And I'm seeing real shifts in my life! My mind is less anxious. I have less judgment and more space to just be me.

I nod my head. "Okay."

"How psychic are you?"

"What do you mean?"

"Are you aware of other people's thoughts and emotions?"

"Ummm . . ." I don't know what to say. I'm not sure what she's talking about . . .

"Lauren, how often have we talked about you taking on other people's pain? Being so empathetic that you actually energetically suck the pain out of them?"

I nod my head again. "Right. I do that. A lot. I've been like that since I was a teenager. My mom called me a sponge. I was like a magnet for people who needed help. I would suck all the yuck out of them, then I would be upset. That was part of the problem when I went crazy. It was too much for me."

"So wouldn't you say that's a form of being psychic and aware?"

"I guess so . . ."

"Okay. Now let's look at your work. When you're at the hospital and feel sad, does that sadness actually belong to you? Is it yours or are you aware of everyone else's sadness?"

This time, rather than trying to figure out the answer to her questions, I remember the Light and Heavy Tool and how the "answer" is in the energy around and in me. I sense a lot of lightness with her questions.

"Wow. It's not mine. None of that sadness is. I just never thought of it as being psychic." I sit there for a few moments in silence. I've seen tons of signs all around San Francisco that say, 'Psychic Reader.'

"I thought psychics read crystal balls."

"You mean you thought psychics were kind of weird and wacky?"

"Yeah I guess so. I never wanted to be weird like that. And nobody ever talked like this with me when I was younger. They all thought I was crazy because I was aware of all of this stuff. They thought it was mania, depression and imbalance. But what you're saying is . . . this is actually my awareness of other people?"

"Yes. This is you being able to know what is going on with other people, and sensing it in your own body and mind. That's all it is. But because you didn't know what it was or how to do anything with it, you got overwhelmed. It's like a radio being tuned in at every single station at one time, and you didn't know what to do with all of that information."

"This is making so much sense to me. It sucks that I didn't have this information when I was younger. It would have changed a lot for me."

I gaze at my hands in my lap, remembering the hundreds of times I sat in doctors' offices with my hands curled up tight in my lap. I lean back into the couch and cross my arms over my chest, giving myself a mini-hug. I close my eyes and take a few deep breaths. I open my eyes again and look Dr. P right in the eyes.

"So I'm not crazy. . . I'm actually psychic? What can I do to not be a sponge and soak up all their sadness and other stuff? How can I still have awareness of their pain but not take on their pain?"

"Here's what you do. It's really simple. The next time you're at work—or really anywhere—but we'll focus on the hospital right now and the sadness. The next time you notice that heavy sensation of the sadness ask the questions, 'Who does this belong to?' 'Is it mine?' Then feel into the energy. If it is heavy then it isn't yours. Then ask 'Is it someone else's?' If it's light then it belongs to them. This allows you to start being aware of what is yours and what is other people's that you are just aware of."

"Is it mine or someone else's?"

"Yes. Exactly. Now here is the cool thing. You don't need to know exactly who it belongs to. You may have an awareness of who it belongs to or not."

"Okay, so if it isn't mine and it is someone else's: then what?"

"And then all you need to do is say, 'Return to Sender.' This lets the Universe know that YOU know it isn't yours and you're not going to hold onto it anymore. Instead, you are returning it to the person it does belong to. The energy is consciousness and knows where to go." She looks at me for a moment to see that I've got it before continuing on.

"You're still going to be aware of the energy of sadness since the people and the environment is still sad but you won't get stuck with thinking it's yours anymore. This way, you can begin to inhabit your own body and your own lightness rather than being so sopping wet like that sponge you described earlier!"

"Mmmm . . . that would be really nice. Wow. I don't know what it would be like to be at the hospital without taking on all of that crap! Is that really possible?"

Dr. P smiles at me, "It does seem strange, doesn't it? Yes, it is possible. And no, you are not crazy: you are psychic; you just haven't known how to tune your radio to your own station! This will really help you do that. So are you willing to try it?"

I smile at her as I stretch my arms up overhead and say, "Yes! No more heavy sponge! Let's return all that crap to sender!"

IT'S NOT MINE!

WHAT'S GOING ON? I look up from where I've been hunched over at the nursing station, writing notes in a patient's chart. I feel like I'm being squashed from all sides. What is this? I felt so light and happy when I stepped into the hospital this morning. But now I feel so tired. And what is this pressure I'm feeling?

I look over at the two nurses who are both staring at their computer screens and typing. A doctor stands a few feet away from me, making what are probably illegible notes in a patient's chart. I return my attention to the chart and continue writing notes. The pressure becomes unbearable. Why do I feel so sad? Dr. P's face flashes before me and I remember the new tool I learned in our last session. Right! This probably isn't even my sadness!

"Who does this belong to?" I ask silently.

"Is it mine?" The space in and around my body gets heavy. No. It's not mine.

"Is it someone else's?" I notice the pressure lifting. I feel a bit lighter.

I see an image of my patient's wife: how she cried as the doctors told her that her husband was at the end of his life and that there was no more we could do. I see the look in my patient's eyes as he desperately tried to communicate his last wishes to his family and the medical team through me, the liaison, the speech therapist.

This sadness is theirs. It is *not* mine. *"Return to sender,"* I say silently.

More lightness. Before I have a moment to enjoy this new lightness, Craig, another speech therapist, comes and leans against the counter, grabbing my arm.

"Lauren! You will not believe what just happened! Those nurses are still not following our recommendations for Room 253!" He lets go of my arm and continues to rant. As he talks I feel a wave of static run up my arm and buzz around in my brain.

"I can't believe that!" The static intensifies.

"I know! I'm going to go talk with the charge nurse!" Craig turns around and leaves.

My heart is beating fast. My face feels flushed. Wait a second . . . What was that, a drive-by annoyance delivery?

"Who does this belong to?" I ask myself again silently. This annoyance and buzzing isn't mine. It's Craig's. It may even belong to the nurses or the patient! It's definitely not mine. *"Return to sender,"* I command silently.

The pounding in my chest slows and the buzzing in my brains stops. I smile as I feel the lightness restored in my body. I don't need to take on this annoyance.

I close my eyes for a moment and beam a message of gratitude to Dr. P. What a gift this is. I just cleared so much heaviness and discomfort with a simple question and command.

I remember a few months ago I got so overwhelmed by all the different energies at the mall. I sat down in the middle of all the hustle and bustle and meditated for thirty minutes before I could do anything, even leave! And even after meditating I felt the heaviness of people's energies. I just didn't realize at the time that none of it was mine!

I jot down a few more notes in the patient's chart and hand it over to one of the nurses. Smiling, I head down the hall to check in with my next patient. As I pass by open doorways I sense different waves of emotions pouring out.

"Nope. I'm not sucking you in anymore. I see you're there but you're not mine to soak in." The power of three little words: Return to Sender. My new best friends!

15

New Possibilities

COMING HOME

"IF YOU COULD HAVE anything out of this session what would it be?" asks Dr. Dain Heer, the Co-Founder of Access Consciousness. I can't believe I'm here, standing next to him, in an Access Consciousness class! After working with Dr. P this past year and learning some Access tools from her, I decided to dive in and start taking some classes myself.

I look at the two other women in our small group. We're in the back of the room getting ready for our special session with Dr. Dain. Behind me I can hear Gary Douglas, the Founder of Access Consciousness, answering one of the other class participant's questions. Even though there are over 100 people in the room, I feel like we're in our own special bubble back here.

I lean against the massage table that I'll be lying on in a moment. Dr. Dain is going to work on all three of us at once. He has his own special blend of healing work that I've never seen before. I've been watching him work on people all weekend, but I still have no idea what to expect.

I scratch my arm as I try to figure out the perfect answer to his question. What should I ask for? What do I want?

The woman on my right speaks first. "I have all these walls up around me. I don't trust people. I'd like to open up more."

The woman across from me says, "I'd like to feel my body more. I've only worked with you once but your touch was so kind. I've never been treated that kindly before. I'd like my body to know more kindness is possible."

Dr. Dain looks over at me and smiles; one eyebrow lifts up as a question to me. All my panic dissolves as I look into his green eyes. In that moment I know what to ask for. "I really liked what she said about being in her body more. Even though I've been doing yoga for years, I still live in my head. I experience brief moments of being in my body and sensations . . . " I pause as I remember the moonlight bath in Peru, the wind on my skin; how I feel in some of my yoga sessions . . . "Most of the time I can't feel my body below my neck though. I would like that to change."

Dr. Dain takes a step back and scans my body. My cheeks get hot. I know he isn't looking just at my physical body; I can tell he is looking deeper, energetically. I wish I knew what he sees.

"Okay," he says. "Go ahead and pick a table and lie face down."

I slip off my black pumps and lie face down. I try to relax and invite my usual meditative state to envelope me. I feel Dr. Dain's hand on my back and then: zppppppppp. A wave of what feels like electricity shoots through my body. I feel like I just got hit with a lightning bolt. Wow. What was that?

Now his hand is on my lower back. Zapppppppp. Zpppppp. Bolt after bolt moves through me. I shudder. I release. The pillow is soaked with my tears. Where is this coming from? I wonder, but I don't stop it. The lightning bolts fade and a wave of calm spreads through my body. My legs and arms tingle with the after effects.

I become aware of the women on the tables near me. I feel a stirring in the air. Even though it's quiet, there is a lot happening in the stillness. I sense the woman closest to me. Is she going to experience her own storm now?

Dr. Dain's hand leaves my lower back and moves to her. Although my eyes are closed, I can sense Dr. Dain touching her feet; I feel it in my own feet as they begin to heat up. My feet! I feel my feet!

I sense waves of energy moving from Dr. Dain to the woman next to me, to me, and to the other woman. My back arches and my legs rise up as I'm lifted by one of these waves. I can feel the woman near me arching up on her table, too. What are these waves we are riding? How is Dr. Dain doing this? My body is coming alive.

The velvet stillness wraps itself around me. As I lie there, now quiet and still, I feel my heart beating. Thump, thump, thump, like a single drumbeat over and over again. The sensation fills me up. And then it's outside of me and inside of me at the same time. Thump, thump, thump; sending little shivers up and down my skin.

It's not just my heartbeat . . . it's all of us. I sense all three of us women and Dr. Dain breathing and beating to the same drum, our breath and hearts synchronizing with one another and with something that is beyond all of us.

More tears flow. I am no longer an empty shell. *"Welcome home,"* I hear. *"Welcome home."*

BUBBLES OF PLEASURE

I'VE BEEN BUZZING EVER since my session with Dr. Dain, and now the entire room is going to have a session with him all at once! What kind of lightning bolts will there be with all of us lying on our backs on the floor?

Two other class participants, Stephanie and Rhonda, come lie down next to me. We've spent the last four days listening to Gary talk about everything from money to relationships to creating our lives. I feel an excitement and eagerness for my life and future that I've never felt before.

I take a deep breath and close my eyes as Dr. Dain's voice fills the large ballroom. I breathe in through my toes and out my head as he suggests and relax into the floor. I hear laughter from a far corner. Dr. Dain continues to talk in a strong yet soothing voice as he walks around the room.

I anticipate another storm of lightning bolts, but they don't come today. Instead, I become aware of a gentle pulse that moves in waves up and down my body. Up and down, up and down, the waves glide over my body, tickling and stroking me with every movement. And then, the waves of energy begin to lap around only one place: my pelvis.

I remember the rakshasa emerging from my pelvis at the meditation retreat. Is that dark energy still there? But this fear dissolves with the next wave that flows over me. Wave after wave of energy sweeps over my pelvis and lower belly, calming, soothing and opening me.

The waves begin to flow faster and faster, just like in the ocean where there are bigger sets of waves. My pelvic muscles contract with such intensity I gasp loudly. I know this energy! It's an orgasm! When was the last time this occurred?

I laugh out loud. The energy slides in waves throughout my body, filling and opening me simultaneously. I melt into the floor. What in the world? Before I have a chance to make sense of this, my pelvis begins to rock.

Again?

Again.

I lose track of time. I lose track of contractions. I lose track of how many times the waves break into a climax.

Somewhere, at some point, the group session with Dr. Dain ends. I can hear people standing up and leaving the room to go to lunch. But my body is still riding the waves as my pelvis contracts and releases.

Although my eyes are closed, I can feel Stephanie and Rhoda's eyes on me. My cheeks flush. I recognize the heat of shame. Here I am lying on the floor having orgasm after orgasm while people move about around me. Who does that? Who is this person? And then the waves in my pelvis push out the shame as though to say: NO. We will not tolerate you anymore.

I cry out and arch up off the floor as another wave moves through me. I run my hands through my hair and moan. "That's beautiful!" I hear Rhonda exclaim. The waves continue. My pelvis responds. One orgasm after another floods me with energy and pleasure.

I sense Stephanie and Rhonda get up to leave. My mind follows them. I turn on my side to get up too but am unable to stand as another contraction in my pelvis takes control. After that wave passes I pull myself up and stumble to a nearby chair, sitting down and doubling over in another wave of pleasure.

"Are you okay?" Dr. Dain asks, gently placing his hand on my shoulder.

"I can't stop coming! I started having orgasms half way through and they won't stop!"

"How does it get any better than that?" Dr. Dain smiles at me.

"What do I do?"

"Enjoy it?"

"Yes. But I can barely walk."

"Lauren, you have control over every energy in your body. Every energy. When you have had enough, ask it to stop. Although, I don't know why you would . . . " he trails off as he moves to check on another class participant.

I have control over every energy in my body. Me. Control. I am in control. I can ask it to stop. Another wave moves through me and I climax, sitting and shuddering in the chair. Control. Surrender. Control.

I'm in the driver's seat here. I can stop this when I want to. It won't drown me; not like when I was a teenager and the energy of everything was overwhelming and out of my control. I get to choose. Do I want it to stop? Not all the way. But I'd like to be able to walk.

My pelvis pulsates with energy, but its insistent pulling lessens as I ask the question and express what I would like. I take a deep breath and stand up slowly. My legs shake and I stumble a little. Slowly, using the chairs for support, I move to the back of the room.

What do you want, body? I ask. Food? No. I don't want to be with people. I'm not hungry. I spot the massage tables and know what I want. I make my way over and crawl onto one of the tables, covering myself with a blanket.

As I lie on my side, the waves slow down. The orgasms stop; my pelvis vibrates with aliveness. Little bubbles of pleasure pop and fade as I dissolve into space.

LIFE IS DIFFERENT NOW

I DANCE AROUND MY apartment, enjoying the soft gray carpet tickling my feet. I pause and balance on my left leg, lifting my right knee up and rotating my right hip in circles.

I hear Elsa meow and turn to see her sauntering towards me. As she rubs up against my left leg I drop my right leg and reach down to stroke her. I move slowly over her fur, feeling past the silkiness, through her skin, past her muscles and bones. Her energy radiates in warmth in the palm of my hand.

I curl myself into a seat next to her and she lies down against my leg. As I place my hands on her belly, the warmth returns to my palms and spreads up my arms and into my chest. It matches the same warmth that is in my pelvis, the same sensation since that class. It hasn't left.

I continue to stroke Elsa. Life is different after that class. My body is giving me information in strange and interesting ways. It seems to be giving information to other people too. It's as though my body and I are partners now, both working to achieve something.

Like with my patient, Mr. F. He hadn't been responding to speech therapy sessions before the class. His voice was tight and his speech was so slurred that I could barely hear him, let alone understand him. Until our session today. . .

At the beginning of our session I uncrossed and then recrossed my legs underneath the therapy table. The sensation of the soft fabric brushing my skin heightened my awareness of my body. I sensed the same thing happened for Mr. F. He sat up straighter in his wheelchair and became more alert.

I wondered what my body was telling me. I silently invited Mr. F to consider his body, too. What's your body telling you? I sensed a relaxing of his muscles all the way from his own leg to his throat.

"I feel better. What was that?" He asked, his voice breaking free from its tightness. The usual scratchiness took on a velvety quality.

"Wow. Listen to that! Yes. Something did change. What's different?"

"I got relaxed. My throat feels more open."

"Cool. Maybe that is something to practice. Where's your awareness when you are talking?"

I feel my lips and tongue more as I ask this and sense his awareness go to his own mouth.

"Oh. I forgot about that. How do I sound now?" He says with clearer articulation.

"How do you think you sound?" I ask, smiling.

"Pretty darn good. Yes, pretty darn good."

Elsa meows again, and I'm back in the room with her. I continue to stroke Elsa as I glance up at the digital clock: 11:36 pm shines at me with a red glow. Wow. It's late.

Oh, wow! I forgot about my weeknight ritual! The one that has been finely honed and followed daily over the past few years. The one that helped me get off meds with my self-management skills.

Home straight away. Shower immediately to wash the hospital dirt and emotional yuck off me. Sit for meditation to cleanse my consciousness. Yoga to ground myself. Television to drown out the noise of life. Turn off TV by 9:00 so I can fall asleep by 10:00. All so I can get up the next day and start all over again.

I didn't do any of this last night nor tonight. I actually forgot about it last night, when the girls at work invited me out for a hike and dinner. And then with tonight's spontaneous dancing, I totally forgot.

I pause to look for any signs of trouble. Am I exhausted by the late hour and gallivanting from last night? Nope. I'm not tired or wired. I just feel good. Am I stressed with the missing of my meditation? Nope. I'm quite relaxed. Am I covered with emotional yuck from the hospital since I missed my cleansing shower? Nope. All's well. Am I ungrounded without my nightly yoga poses? Nope. I look down at my feet and wiggle my toes. I can still feel them. Hmmm . . .

I had fun tonight. I broke the self-care ritual. Nothing bad happened. Dr. S's voice rings in my head, *"I think you can manage yourself with your yoga, diet and lifestyle."* Wouldn't she be surprised to see me like this? Calm, happy and having fun with no ritual. Yes. Life is different after that class. Maybe it's time to loosen the reins and see what else is possible.

CAGED ANIMAL

I PACE ALONG THE dirt path like a caged animal, looking for a way out. For the past four days I've walked this same short route from the retreat center to the closed gate, back and forth and back and forth. I'm surprised there aren't grooves in the dirt from my footsteps.

I reach the gate at the edge of the retreat center grounds and stare out at the Costa Rican lushness. I want *out!* I want to *move!* I sigh loudly and shake my shoulders. Nothing has changed since yesterday. The path hasn't gotten any longer. The gate is still closed. Only my energy is building. I turn away from the gate and walk among the biggest trees I've ever seen.

Usually I enjoy the smallness I feel being amidst these giants. But today I feel as tall as the trees. My arms could be their limbs, stretching up into the bright blue sky. My chest is strong, like their trunks, thumping with life. My legs though—my legs are moving, carrying me along the trail with quick steps. No rootedness there.

The air around me vibrates with insects buzzing. Everything is pulsing. Connected. Vibrant. Electric. Bubbles flow through me, zipping and zapping with the moss, the orchids, the trees.

Goose bumps shiver up and down my arms even though it's muggy. I feel like I did that day, before I was diagnosed with bipolar, when I had to leave the house for fear I would make it explode with all my energy.

I begin to feel the earth beating with me. Thump-thump-thump. I move faster and start to skip, trying to move the energy that is building up inside of me.

Agh! I come to an abrupt halt and stare out past the gate again at the twisty road and lush green forest. I see a road sign: it's in Spanish. I know there are hiking trails out there but I can't read the map with directions for how to find them. Is it safe out there? What if I get lost? I don't speak the language.

I look at my watch. Four minutes! That's it? I whip around and look down the trail I've just walked at least five times. This is the first time I timed myself. It took me four minutes to walk this stretch of trail from the classroom to the gate.

I jump up and down. I want *out!* I shake my arms and legs as I gaze out beyond the gate again. I remember my parents telling me not to cross the bridge into the woods beyond our neighborhood when I went for daily walks after my diagnosis. They were afraid for me. They didn't think I should go that far. Yet I disobeyed them. Where is that courage now?

Arghhh! I turn around and fly down the path, skipping in big arcs, up and down, back and forth on the trail. Is this what a tiger feels like, locked in a cage?

I've been here in Costa Rica for five days already. This Access Consciousness class is like nothing I've ever experienced before. Being immersed in these tools and teachings, day after day, in the midst of so much beauty and pulsating life, has stirred me up. All that energy, all those bubbles, are emerging at an accelerated rate. They are stretching the space between my bones and my skin.

I arrive at the gate again and stand there, staring at the latch. I scratch my arms. I look out past the gate into the green space that seems to be calling my name, beckoning me, reaching its arms out to me, inviting me to come forward. I reach out and touch the metal latch. It's warm and inviting. Before I can lift it, I hear my name being called. "Lauren? Hey Lauren: we're heading back to class. Break is over."

The wild open space beyond the gate is calling me to go forward. But I pull my hand back from the latch. "Not today," I mutter, gazing out for another moment before turning and heading up the trail to class.

BREAKING FREE

THE BRIGHT SUNLIGHT DAZZLES my eyes as I step outside the classroom. I blink several times, adjusting to the light after seven days of cloudy skies. I raise my face to the sun and its warmth kisses my face.

I head towards the short path that's been my "hiking trail" this week. As I enter the forest I notice the quiet. I pause and listen. My mind is absolutely still. No chatter. And not only that, the bubbles that were zapping me the other day are flowing, not bursting with electricity.

I hear the insects and sounds of the forest, but now there is a calm to them that is new. Or perhaps it was always there and now I can perceive it? As I move down the path towards the gate I feel carried by a wave of bubbles, as if a soft breeze is pressing into my back, both moving me forward and lifting me up at the same time.

I look up at the trees and their canopy of branches that spread out above me. Today I am expansive but they still tower over me. I pause and lift my arms up overhead, swaying back and forth like their branches. Immediately I sense a wave of bubbles spreading up to the trees, connecting me to them and them to me. I become taller as I commune with them.

"You have control over every energy in your body," I hear Dr. Dain's voice in my head, *"Every energy."*

I've been playing with the bubbles and electricity that have been buzzing through me these past few days. I was letting them take control of me, fearing their intensity. It's all energy, I keep telling myself. It's all energy, and I get to control it. It can't override me. It can't take me over like it used to when I was a teenager.

I know now how to use tools like, "Who does this belong to?" and "Return to sender". I know when the energy is mine and is inviting me to receive and ride it.

I discovered I don't need to harness the energy; yes, I can control it, but that doesn't mean I need to push it down. It's like I finally have a finger on the volume dial and can adjust it to where I like it, ten seconds at a time.

Yesterday I found the courage to go beyond the gate with two other women from the class. Why was it easier to go with them? Why didn't I have the courage to go beyond the gate before that, on my own? My self-judgments fade as I say out loud, "What else is possible?"

I move towards the gate, picking up my pace. Today I'm ready to go through the gate on my own. Today the gate isn't an obstacle: it's an invitation. As I near it something catches my eye. All I can see and sense is movement. What is that?

I reach the gate and gasp. Horses! Brown, white and black horses are milling about. I try to count them but they keep moving and it's hard to track them. Ten? Twelve? I don't see any people and the horses don't have any bridles on. Where did they come from?

I reach down and pull up on the latch, stepping through and into the open space beyond. I breathe in deeply and stare at the horses as I close the gate behind me. They are beautiful. I move down the road to them, watching as they nibble on grass and rub up against each other.

"They are quite something, aren't they?" The unexpected voice startles me from behind, I turn and see a young woman and two young girls.

"They are! Where did they all come from?"

"They're from different homes around here."

"They aren't being supervised by anyone?"

"No. People let them wander in the middle of the day. They are headed to that meadow on the right where they'll eat and hang out with each other. And then at night they'll return home."

She smiles at me as I take this in: horses being left to wander; their owners trusting them to return at night; and the horses choosing to return to closed quarters!

I turn my attention to the girls. "Do you live here?"

"Yes," the taller one answers quietly, looking up to meet my eyes and then looking over at the horses again.

I smile at her, "You sound American."

"We moved here a few years ago," the mother replies for the girl who is mesmerized by the horses. "It's been quite amazing and very different from the States. Are you staying at the retreat center?"

"Yes, I'm here for a week."

"Oh, lucky you."

I nod my head in agreement and then we both turn our attention to the horses. What would it be like to ride one of them as they wander these curvy roads? To sit on the back of one of these powerful creatures and allow it to carry me anywhere?

"Mommy, I'm ready to go." The youngest girl pulls on her mother's skirt, tugging for the return of her mother's attention.

"Okay," the mother says to the girl, taking her hand. "It was nice meeting you. Enjoy your retreat!"

"You too, and thank you." I watch the three of them head down the road, moving in between the horses. The youngest girl turns and waves goodbye.

As they disappear around a curve I watch the entire herd of horses—fifteen! I count—move into the meadow, just as the woman said they would.

That's when it dawns on me . . . I am beyond the gate! And like the horses, I am free to roam. The wave of bubbles returns and pushes me forward, gently. I head down the road in the opposite direction from the woman and her two girls.

I reach a fork in the road. Yesterday we turned left here. That led to houses and cars. I don't want that today. I look to the right and see lush, wild jungle. That's what I want. I turn right and keep walking.

The rumble of a car startles me. I freeze: both my body and my breath hold still. I look and see a truck full of men coming in my direction. I hear my dad's voice, *"Don't go wandering alone. It's not safe for a woman."*

The bubbles in my belly crash into each other. I move over to the side of the narrow road. I force myself to breathe. Relax, I tell myself. Relax. It's okay. The men wave and smile at me as they pass. The truck doesn't even slow down. I laugh out loud. I'm safe.

I peel off my sweater and feel the wind on my skin. I start walking again. I come to a fork in the road. Right or left? Backwards or forwards? I get to choose. Ten seconds at a time. I've got the reins! I choose left, moving forward, swiveling my hips from side to side as I go.

ROSE GARDEN

THE ROSES GREET ME as I step out of the rehabilitation department and walk along the path towards the hospital. I lift my face to the early morning sun and take several deep breaths, luxuriating in their sweet scent.

I slow my steps. Yes, there is a lot to do today, a lot of patients to see, but I don't have to rush. I move through the rose garden, enjoying the mini-rainbows that are created as the sun sparkles in the dewdrops. There are red, white and pink blossoms. I bend to touch their soft petals. No. No need to rush: that won't make the day move faster, me more productive or help me serve my patients better.

"Stopping to smell the roses, eh, Lauren?" one of the custodians comments as he passes by. I smile and nod at him.

"Glad to see you so calm and happy, as always," he winks at me and moves ahead at a quicker pace.

"Who would have thought?" I whisper to the roses, "Me, calm and happy, at the hospital!"

How many of the patients and staff have expressed comments like this to me over the past several months? The staff was so curious to know my tricks for being calm amidst all the stress of the hospital that they asked me to offer a class. ME! Me, who used to be overwhelmed by too much noise and mayhem! Who would have thought?

As I move towards the hospital doors, I remember the look on their faces as I shared the simple techniques they could use to clear away overwhelm and enjoy their experience at the hospital. Their faces filled with awe as they put the tools I shared into practice and saw the benefits themselves.

I push open the double doors and head down the hallway to the I.C.U. I notice the air is different here; no rose scent, it's stale and dense with a combination of sadness and stress. But the rose fragrance clings to my nostrils and the density doesn't weigh me down. I'm aware none of it is mine.

I pass the doors to the E.R. and feel like I've been punched in the gut. I start to walk faster. I catch myself, slow down, breathe deeply and say, "Return to Sender," silently. That stress and urgency is not mine.

"Morning, Lauren!" Maria calls out to me from behind the radiology registration desk. "I see we have two swallow studies today. You have a busy morning!"

"Yes. I'll be back soon to do them. I'm headed to the I.C.U. first for a stat patient." I smile at her as I walk past the desk. Her rosy cheeks remind me of the pink roses in the garden.

I round the corner and stop short of a doctor. "Good! You are here early. Are you going to see the patient in 3D2?" his words come out in one long string, as though he can't get them out fast enough. I pause before answering, take a deep breath and look him in the eye. "Yep. That's where I'm headed now."

I deliberately slow my pace as I move away from him. No need to rush, I remind myself. It's not going to help anyone. No need to let others' stress affect me. As I move through the unit, staff call out to me in cheerful greetings or rushed urgency. Patients cry in pain, call out in hallucination or smile at my familiar face as I pass by.

I continue to move forward down the hallway just like I did along the path through the rose garden. Why does walking through the hospital need to be any different?

I'VE COME A LONG WAY

A SIGH ESCAPES MY lips as I drop my backpack onto the floor and sink into a cushioned seat at Gate 32. A man nearby looks up at me with a scowl. "Sorry!" I say to him with a smile,

"My backpack is heavy. It feels so good to take it off!" His scowl softens into a smile as he returns to reading his paper.

I rub my shoulders and lean back into the seat. I gaze out the windows at the airplanes coming and going. Beyond them I see the wide expanse of the Norwegian countryside. Oslo is so beautiful. How did I get so lucky?

I can't help but bask in the glow of these past two weeks. Facilitating nine days of classes. A half-dozen private sessions. In all of them I have seen people discover more of themselves. As they gave up the idea that there was something wrong with them and instead, started to see their greatness, their eyes sparkled with tears, joy and possibility.

I hug myself and almost laugh out loud as I remember going skinny-dipping during lunchtime one day. While the class participants were eating I slipped away for a dip in the freezing cold water of the North Sea. I skipped from rock to rock, luxuriating in the feel of the warm sun and cold water.

"Miss?" I look up to see the ticket agent hovering above me. "Yes?"

"You are all set," she says, handing me a slip of paper, "Thank you for volunteering to give up your seat on this flight. Here is your $700 voucher."

A 700-dollar flight voucher! This will help cover my flight to Geneva in two months where I'll be teaching more classes.

"I'm going to escort you to your next flight. We have to move quickly if you are going to catch it. Please follow me."

I take the paper from her and slip it into my backpack. "Are we in a time crunch?" I ask as I pick up my backpack and sling it over my shoulder.

"Yes. The next flight leaves sooner than this one and we have to get your suitcase and check it on the new airline."

She turns and leads the way to the other gate. Her hurried steps and rushed speech remind me of the hospital. I notice my own steps start to quicken and then I stop myself. Nope, I'm not going there, especially after this amazing experience. I slow my pace and focus on breathing deeply.

The flight attendant continues ahead. She stops and looks over her shoulder at me, several steps behind her. I smile at her.

"Oh, you're back there. I'm moving too fast!"

"I just don't like rushing," I say. "It makes me more stressed than needed."

"That's true," she says and waits for me to catch up with her. As we begin to move together she matches my long steady stride.

"How long have you worked for the airline?" I ask her. She smiles and visibly relaxes as she shares her story with me. We collect my luggage from baggage claim and begin to make our way to the other gate.

As we move through the airport, people swirl around us like a tornado. I used to hate crowds; now I breathe deeply, deliberately keep my pace steady, and weave through the crowd. I smile wider. I feel like the calm in the storm.

Bubbles release from my pelvis but instead of exploding, I expand them. I become the space and lightness of the bubbles. They don't pop or burst. I don't need to shove them down or control them. I allow them to get bigger than the tornado. I become the space that is bigger than the storm.

I glide behind my personal ticket agent as she cuts the line to check my bag for me. Then she guides me quickly through security. We arrive at the gate right as it begins boarding. She smiles broadly at me as she hands me my boarding pass.

"Wow! That was perfect timing," she says.

"Yes. Yes, it was," I smile at her surprised expression and turn to join the line of waiting passengers, breathing deeply into the expanded bubble of lightness I am.

A FINAL NOTE TO YOU, DEAR READER...

RECEIVING A DIAGNOSIS of "bipolar" put me in a box. All the doctors and experts had answers and different perspectives about how to manage my bipolar "problem." They were all sources of information *outside of myself.* They were helpful at the time but I knew there was something more . . .

I knew I didn't belong in a box. None of us do. Labels are limitations. They are definitions used to categorize people in a broad way. They do not take individual uniqueness into consideration. Allowing labels to define who you are and who you will be is one of the most destructive things you can do.

Throughout this book, I have mentioned tools that have helped me create the changes I desired in my life. As I used these tools I discovered that what I had always considered as my wrongness, my craziness, was actually a unique set of gifts and capacities that nobody—including myself—had understood. There was nothing ever wrong with me. There is nothing ever wrong with any of us. We are each unique and just require tools and self-awareness to use our gifts in generative ways.

Now I travel around the world, guiding others on the path of transforming their "wrongness" into their "strongness" and sharing tools they can use to create new lives for themselves. To help recall these tools, refer to the Resource section. Keep in mind: there is no one way to do anything. That includes healing yourself, being in this world or creating a life that works for you.

We all have gifts and capacities. We all have differences. We get to educate ourselves on what those are and how to use them for our greatest enjoyment and contribution to the world. This journey will look different for each of us.

As I shared with you in the beginning of the book:

I am here to let you know there is a possibility for your life far beyond what you can see right now. There is freedom from this pain.

I have shared with you the journey I took to discover the other side of bipolar, beyond the lies and limitation of mental illness. There are other possibilities available to you now, too.

Will you choose to go beyond the label or other limitation that has you trapped in a box?

What else is possible for you when you let go of your wrongness and discover it as your strongness?

My biggest wish for you is that you allow yourself to explore your unique gifts and perception of the world.

The world needs your difference. Are you willing to be it?

With all that I am,
Lauren Polly

RESOURCES

Tools for Moving Beyond "Difference" as a "Disability"

THESE ARE THE TOOLS that I used on my journey and mentioned in this book. May they support you, as they did me, to move beyond labels, limitations and what others think of you.

DIET, REST AND EXERCISE: Eat foods that make you feel spacious. Get as much rest as needed. Move your body daily in any way that feels fun. When you tune into your body and give it what it requires, you get out of the anxious and depressed mind and discover more of the resources and awareness that your body has.

ENVISION A FUTURE YOU DESIRE: Get clear on what you would like your future to be like. If there were no limitations, no roadblocks and no reasons why you couldn't be or do or have something—what would you choose to be, do and have as your future?

SCRAPBOOKING: Play with poems, quotes, journaling, artwork and anything else that allows you to reflect on the past, make peace with the present and start to dream about the future.

JOURNALING: This allows you a private outlet to rant, dream, reveal and get clarity on your day-to-day life.

ALTERNATIVE FORMS OF THERAPY: Art, dance or theater therapies are powerful modalities for self-expression, release and building confidence.

YOGA: Yoga means "union," and it invites you into communion with your body and being. Experiencing yoga on and off the mat can cultivate inner calm and a sense of spacious possibilities.

MEDITATION: There are many different kinds of meditation yet the benefits are similar: quiet the mind, experience more presence in the moment and discover a sense of peace and calm.

NEURO EMOTIONAL TECHNIQUE®: NET is a mind-body technique that finds and removes neurological imbalances related to unresolved stress. To find a practitioner visit: netmind-body.com/find-a-practitioner

PAST LIFE AWARENESS: We often have deeply ingrained reactionary patterns based on our past lives. This technique can facilitate you getting free of the reactions while tapping into the gifts of these past life awarenesses.

ACCESS CONSCIOUSNESS®: A wide array of pragmatic tools, new perspectives and hands on energy work that guide you to access your consciousness through self-empowerment, curiosity and non-judgment. (www.accessconsciousness.com) The following are tools from Access Consciousness:

- *Asking Questions:* Questions open a space for more possibilities to reveal themselves to you. Don't look for answers. Instead, tune into the energies and awareness that arise after asking a question.

- *Light/Heavy:* One way to tap into energetic awareness and personal knowing is to ask a question and feel into the energy in and around your body. If it is light then it is true for you, if it is heavy then it isn't. This is an amazing tool to start being empowered to know what you know.

- *Who Does This Belong To?:* Most of our thoughts, feelings and emotions aren't ours; we are simply aware of the world and people around us. We get stuck when we personalize our awareness, and believe the thoughts, feelings and emotions we are experiencing are ours. By asking, "Who does this belong to?" and tuning into what's light and what's heavy, we discover what is really ours and what belongs to someone else. This tool can help you—like it helped me— find yourself amidst the noise of the world.

About the Author

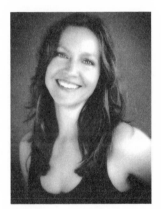

LAUREN POLLY is a catalyst for people who are living their life on autopilot. Through her cutting-edge classes and 1:1 coaching, she's able to help you shift from surviving to thriving through dynamic healing, self-empowerment, and life-changing tools.

Her practical and light-hearted teachings are featured in *The Change 6: Insights into Self-Empowerment* (Jim Britt & Jim Lutes, 2015), and on her weekly radio show, *Beyond Speech, Limitless Communication*.

A Certified Access Consciousness® Facilitator, Certified Talk to the Entities® Facilitator, ASHA Certified Medical Speech-Language Pathologist and Registered Yoga Instructor, Lauren has shown thousands of people around the world how to engage boldly with themselves, their body and the world, so they create the life they desire.

Meet Lauren and be inspired at www.LaurenPolly.com.

Lauren Polly's Workshops

ACCESS BARS®

THE BARS ARE 32 POINTS on the head that, when touched lightly, start to clear out all limitations you have about different areas of your life and your body. This leads to relaxation, stress relief and more possibilities! In this 1-day class you will learn the basic tools in Access Consciousness and give and receive 2 Bars sessions, which trains you to give the Bars to others. (8 hours CEU available for massage therapists)

ACCESS FOUNDATION®

IN THIS CLASS YOU begin to undo the limitations you've been functioning from and establish the foundation for creating a different reality. You will begin to see the points of view that limit you and what you can change that would allow you to function from a more conscious space, where you are no longer at the effect of this reality. This class provides hundreds of tools, including some hands-on body processes, that allow you to change anything that isn't working for you in your life.

TALK TO THE ENTITIES®

TALK TO THE ENTITIES is a fully comprehensive system for learning how to deal with, facilitate, clear, receive from and have overall ease and peace with the spirit world. In these classes you will learn a set of tools, processes and philosophies that will totally revolutionize the way you think, feel and function with the spirit world.

BEING SOCIAL

UNCOVERING THE GRACEFUL YOU. In this workshop you will: find your authenticity of expression, grow adept at dealing with difficult people/circumstances, increase intimacy in personal relations and ease in social interactions, cultivate artful manipulation, discover what works for you when relating to others, expand your creative expression and enjoy more ease, fun and spontaneity with every interaction!

HAPPY BODY HAPPY YOU

DEVELOPING EASE FROM THE INSIDE OUT. In this workshop you will: release body judgments, shift dis-ease to ease, learn how to listen to your body and heighten its sensation and pleasure, create dynamic sexual play and relationships, develop your self-confidence and body love, cultivate living from a relaxed state, know your desires and how to receive them and begin living a happy life in partnership with your body!

MENTAL HEALTH EMPOWERMENT

RECLAIMING YOUR HOPE. In this workshop you will learn real time practical tools to assist daily upsets, build self-awareness to find yourself in the noise of the world, set targets for moving away from destructive behaviors, unlock and re-direct energy towards creative pursuits and build your awareness to trust YOU above all else!

For more information on all of Lauren's classes, visit:
www.laurenpolly.com

To invite Lauren to speak at an event, host her for a workshop or schedule a 1:1 session email:
lauren@laurenpolly.com